MINDFULNESS IN SOCIAL PSYCHOLOGY

Scientific interest in mindfulness has expanded in recent years, but it has typically been approached from a clinical perspective. This volume brings recent mindfulness research to classic social psychology topics such as romantic relationships, prejudice, prosocial behaviour, achievement, and self-control. Written by renowned scholars in social psychology, it combines a comprehensive research overview with an in-depth analysis of the processes through which mindfulness affects people's daily life experiences. It provides theoretical and methodological guidance for researchers across disciplines and discusses fundamental processes in mindfulness, including its effect on emotion regulation, executive control, automatic and deliberative processing, and its relationship to self-construal and self-identity. This book will be of particular interest to upper-level students and researchers in social psychology, health psychology, and clinical psychology, as well as social work and psychology professionals.

Johan C. Karremans is Associate Professor in the Behavioural Science Institute at Radboud University Nijmegen, the Netherlands.

Esther K. Papies is Senior Lecturer in the Institute of Neuroscience and Psychology at the University of Glasgow, United Kingdom.

Current Issues in Social Psychology
Series Editor: Arjan E. R. Bos

Current Issues in Social Psychology is a series of edited books that reflect the state-of-the-art of current and emerging topics of interest in basic and applied social psychology.

Each volume is tightly focused on a particular topic and consists of seven to ten chapters contributed by international experts. The editors of individual volumes are leading figures in their areas and provide an introductory overview.

Example topics include: self-esteem, evolutionary social psychology, minority groups, social neuroscience, cyberbullying, and social stigma.

Power and Identity
Edited by Denis Sindic, Manuela Barret, and Rui Costa-Lopes

Cyberbullying: From Theory to Intervention
Edited by Trijntje Völlink, Francine Dehue, and Conor Mc Guckin

Coping with Lack of Control in a Social World
Edited by Marcin Bukowski, Immo Fritsche, Ana Guinote, and Mirosław Kofta

Intergroup Contact Theory: Recent Developments and Future Directions
Edited by Loris Vezzali & Sofia Stathi

Majority and Minority Influence: Societal Meaning and Cognitive Elaboration
Edited by Stamos Papastamou, Antonis Gardikiotis, and Gerasimos Prodromitis

Mindfulness in Social Psychology
Edited by Johan C. Karremans and Esther K. Papies

MINDFULNESS IN SOCIAL PSYCHOLOGY

Edited by
Johan C. Karremans and Esther K. Papies

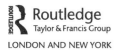

Routledge
Taylor & Francis Group

LONDON AND NEW YORK

First published 2017
by Routledge
2 Park Square, Milton Park, Abingdon, Oxon OX14 4RN

and by Routledge
711 Third Avenue, New York, NY 10017

Routledge is an imprint of the Taylor & Francis Group, an informa business

British Library Cataloguing-in-Publication Data
A catalogue record for this book is available from the British Library

Library of Congress Cataloging-in-Publication Data
Names: Karremans, Johan C., editor. | Papies, Esther K., editor.
Title: Mindfulness in social psychology / edited by Johan C. Karremans and Esther K. Papies.
Description: Abingdon, Oxon ; New York, NY : Routledge, 2017. | Series: Current issues in social psychology | Includes bibliographical references and index.
Identifiers: LCCN 2016052550 | ISBN 9781138646131 (hardback : alk. paper) | ISBN 9781138646148 (pbk. : alk. paper) | ISBN 9781315627700 (ebook)
Subjects: LCSH: Mindfulness (Psychology) | Social psychology.
Classification: LCC BF637.M56 M564 2017 | DDC 302.5/4—dc23
LC record available at https://lccn.loc.gov/2016052550

ISBN: 978-1-138-64613-1 (hbk)
ISBN: 978-1-138-64614-8 (pbk)
ISBN: 978-1-315-62770-0 (ebk)

Typeset in Bembo
by Apex CoVantage, LLC

CONTENTS

CONTRIBUTORS

Hugo J.E.M. Alberts, Maastricht University, The Netherlands

Lawrence W. Barsalou, University of Glasgow, United Kingdom

Daniel R. Berry, Virginia Commonwealth University, United States

Kirk Warren Brown, Virginia Commonwealth University, United States

Paul Condon, Northeastern University, United States

J. David Creswell, Carnegie Mellon University, United States

Kate J. Diebels, Duke University, United States

Nathaniel Elkins-Brown, University of Toronto, Canada

Madeleine E. Gross, University of California Santa Barbara, United States

Michael Inzlicht, University of Toronto, Canada

Gesa Kappen, Radboud University Nijmegen, The Netherlands

Johan C. Karremans, Radboud University Nijmegen, The Netherlands

Mark R. Leary, Duke University, United States

Emily K. Lindsay, Carnegie Mellon University, United States

Alissa J. Mrazek, Northwestern University, United States

Michael D. Mrazek, University of California Santa Barbara, United States

Esther K. Papies, University of Glasgow, United Kingdom

Dawa T. Phillips, University of California Santa Barbara, United States

Hayley Rahl, Carnegie Mellon University, United States

Jonathan W. Schooler, University of California Santa Barbara, United States

Jerry Slutsky, Carnegie Mellon University, United States

Rimma Teper, University of Toronto, Canada

Claire M. Zedelius, University of California Santa Barbara, United States

1

WHY SOCIAL PSYCHOLOGISTS SHOULD CARE ABOUT MINDFULNESS

Johan C. Karremans and Esther K. Papies

Why social psychologists should care about mindfulness

Over the past 30 years, the concept of mindfulness has found its way into main-stream psychological science. Initially, research approached mindfulness mainly from clinical and neurocognitive perspectives, focusing on its potential stress-buffering effects and the prevention and reduction of depressive symptoms. Mindfulness, however, may have much broader implications, and these are increasingly recognized by scientists. As noted by Jon Kabat-Zinn, one of the pioneering scholars in this field, "mindfulness [...] has profound relevance for our present-day lives" (1994, p. 3). Mindfulness not only may impact a general sense of well-being and health, but may affect daily activities like eating, sleeping, and learning; it may affect our emotions, our goals, and the decisions we make; and it may affect our sense of self and how we interact with and relate to other people.

Social psychology is the science of everyday human behaviour, and not surprisingly then, interest in mindfulness has started to increase among social psychologists as well. Yet, while articles on this topic appear regularly in the main social psychology journals, the concept is still studied by only a relatively small subgroup of social psychologists. In this chapter, we reach out to a broader audience and argue that the concept of mindfulness may have important implications for a wide variety of topics that are traditionally studied by social psychologists. We first provide a brief historical background, and we discuss what mindfulness is, and what it is not. Reviewing recent mindfulness research on social psychological topics, we then discuss how social psychology as a field could benefit from engaging with mindfulness for theory, empirical research, and applications. Finally, we will discuss how mindfulness researchers in turn could profit from integrating social psychological theory and methodology into their work. In doing so, we hope to inspire constructive cross-talk between the fields.

A brief history of mindfulness in Western science

The concept of mindfulness was introduced in Western psychology in the late 70s by Jon Kabat-Zinn, a medical scientist at the University of Massachusetts. Rooted in Buddhist contemplative traditions and teachings (for an extensive discussion, see Williams & Kabat-Zinn, 2013), Kabat-Zinn developed a secular mindfulness-training program. Using meditation exercises and psycho-education, participants gradually learn to stabilize their attention to increase moment-to-moment aware-ness of body sensations, thoughts, and emotions, and to approach these experiences non-judgementally and with curiosity. Initially developed to treat patients with chronic pain, over the years a large number of participants around the world have participated in mindfulness-based training programs for a wide variety of reasons, including anxiety, depressive symptoms, and stress; sleeping problems; rumination; impulsivity and aggressive tendencies; concentration problems; or simply for per-sonal and spiritual growth.

In the wake of the growing popularity of these programs in Western society, a first wave of mindfulness research emerged. Clinical studies started to evaluate the effectiveness of the training programs, and of mindfulness meditation practice more generally, for issues such as depression relapse prevention (Teasdale, Segal, & Williams, 1995), the treatment of anxiety disorders (Miller, Fletcher, & Kabat-Zinn, 1995), and quality of life among chronic pain patients (Kabat-Zinn, 1982; Kabat-Zinn, Lipworth, & Burney, 1985). While the evaluation of mindfulness-based inter-ventions with regard to individual health and well-being is still a rapidly expanding field of research, mindfulness-related techniques have already been incorporated into various forms of clinical practice (e.g. acceptance and commitment therapy, mindfulness-based cognitive therapy; see Baer, 2015).

Once support for the effectiveness of mindfulness in promoting psychological well-being had accumulated, a second wave of inquiry – roughly the past 15 years – concentrated on the more specific question of *how* the effects of mindfulness emerge. For example, neuroscientists and cognitive psychologists started to examine the cog-nitive and neural underpinnings of mindfulness, finding evidence that mindfulness is associated with increases in executive control (Teper, Segal, & Inzlicht, 2013; see also Elkins-Brown, Teper, & Inzlicht, Chapter 5 in this volume), attentional control (Chambers, Lo, & Allen, 2008), and structural changes in brain areas associated with such functions (e.g. Davidson et al., 2003; Hölzel et al., 2011; Zeidan et al., 2011). Moreover, as we will discuss in this chapter, researchers began paying increased theo-retical and empirical attention to the specific psychological mechanisms that may be associated with mindfulness, such as changes in emotion regulation and empa-thy (e.g. Goldin & Gross, 2010; Birnie, Speca, & Carlson, 2010, respectively), and changes in perspectives on the self (see Leary & Diebels, Chapter 4 in this volume).

What is mindfulness – and what is it not?

But what exactly *is* mindfulness? Although a variety of definitions have been sug-gested, researchers most commonly define mindfulness as a state of paying conscious

attention to present-moment experiences with an open and non-judgemental attitude (Kabat-Zinn, 1990). In this definition, two components can be distinguished:
1) focusing *attention* on present-moment experiences, including bodily sensations,
thoughts, and emotional states, and 2) approaching these experiences with a *non-
judgemental* attitude, irrespective of their valence (Bishop et al., 2004). Thus, being
mindful means observing one's immediate and current experiences, and acknowledge them for what they are in this present moment, or put differently, giving them
bare attention (Epstein, 2008).[1]

Although this may sound relatively simple and easy to do, most people who
have attempted to train this skill, through meditation or mindfulness training, have
quickly found that it can be quite difficult. While important individual differences exist (see for example Alberts, Chapter 2 in this volume), various domains
of research suggest that for many people a state of mindful awareness is not something that occurs naturally, nor often, in daily life. Some would even say that most
of the time, people are and act in a state of *mindlessness*. For example, research on
automaticity suggests that significant portions of our daily activities are guided by
unconscious and automatic processes (Wyer, 2014). Moreover, the mind has an
extremely strong tendency to wander, and without realizing it, people are typically
engrossed in thoughts about the past or future, rather than the present moment,
relating their experiences to their self-concepts (Farb et al., 2007) and making them
unhappy (Killingsworth & Gilbert, 2010). In addition, as soon as negative emotions
or difficulties occur, many people have an automatic tendency to avoid or suppress
the experience, turning their attention *away* from it (Gross & John, 2003). On top
of this, people often judge, approach, and avoid objects and other people automatically, as social psychologists have convincingly shown (e.g. Chen & Bargh, 1999;
Greenwald & Banaji, 1995; Herring et al., 2013).

All of these examples of mind*less*ness can be contrasted with a state of mindfulness, in which a person attends to and becomes aware of internal experiences and
automatic response tendencies; the mind is not wandering but focused on the present moment; and one is turning attention *towards* experiences – whether negative,
neutral, or positive – receptive to whatever is going on in mind and body, with an
attitude of acceptance and non-judgement. In other words, a state of mindfulness
can be described as a state in which one takes a *decentered* meta-cognitive perspective on one's current-moment experiences, including one's thoughts and feelings
about the self, rather than immediately responding to them (e.g. Bishop et al.,
2004). To give an example: One may observe that, at this very moment, there is an
emotional tone of anger, that there is tension in the body, that there are thoughts
about revenge, and perhaps behavioural inclinations to aggress. Instead of immers-
ing oneself in these experiences, in a mindful state, one's perspective shifts from
"within one's subjective experience onto that experience" (p. 599; Bernstein et al.,
2015), which may fundamentally change how these experiences affect us, and may
provide one with more 'freedom' of how to respond next.

Before we start discussing how this all may be applied to social psychological
theory and research, it is helpful to consider briefly how mindfulness can be distinguished from related concepts, particularly those that have been studied extensively

in social psychology (for a more extensive discussion, see Brown & Ryan, 2003). First, some of these concepts also entail attention and awareness, most notably self-monitoring and self-awareness. *Self-monitoring* refers to the capacity to observe and evaluate one's behaviour against a set of standards or norms (Snyder, 1974), allowing one to adjust one's behaviour accordingly. Relatedly, *self-awareness* refers to the ability to recognize one's feelings, behaviours, and traits, and evaluate and compare them to internal standards (Wicklund, 1975). While there is some overlap of these concepts with mindfulness in that the focus of attention is on internal experiences, mindfulness critically differs from them as it not concerned with standards or norms. It entails the observing of direct experience *not* through an evaluative lens, without trying to understand the experience or having the immediate intention of changing it. Second, while mindfulness requires the regulation of attention, and mindfulness can promote successful self-regulation (see Elkins-Brown et al., Chapter 5 in this volume), it should not be equated with self-regulation or self-control. Whereas self-control entails the active down-regulation of emotions or impulses, mindfulness means to simply observe them as they are, with no other goal than simply observing – even though almost paradoxically, this often facilitates their regulation. Finally, it is important to mention that the concept of mindfulness discussed in this volume differs from Langer's conceptualization of mindfulness (Langer, 1989), which refers to mindfulness as the ability to "notice new things", not determined by old routines or rules, when paying full momentary attention to one's surroundings. While the concepts overlap in the sense that they both entail paying attention with an open and curious mind, the concept of mindfulness we refer to is concerned with non-judgemental, meta-cognitive attention to the nature of one's momentary experiences (not the external world per se).

These differences from self-related concepts typically studied by social psychologists reflect the fact that while psychological research traditionally is concerned with studying the consequences of particular *contents* of consciousness (e.g. certain biases, specific thoughts, specific emotions, and so forth), mindfulness is concerned with the *nature* of people's cognitive processes and experiences, rather than their specific content. As a result, mindfulness as an intervention technique is also distinct from typical emotion regulation techniques like reappraisal, which focus on changing the content of one's thoughts or experiences. Instead, mindfulness is concerned with changing how one perceives and relates to the contents of consciousness (e.g. experiencing them as 'real' vs. accepting them as mere mental events). As will be discussed in greater detail later in this chapter, this can have important implications for how one is affected by and responds to thoughts and emotions.

The value of mindfulness for social psychological research

What is the potential value of studying mindfulness for understanding everyday human behaviour? Why should social psychologists care about mindfulness? We propose that mindfulness is relevant for social psychologists because it has implications for social psychological theory, particularly where automaticity and self-relatedness are concerned, and it has important implications for applications to positively affect people's lives.

Implications for social psychological theory

As noted by Barsalou (Chapter 3 in this volume), mindfulness's distinct focus on *attention* to internal experiences has important consequences for the interplay of automatic and controlled processes. Mindfulness also directly affects self-related processes (e.g. Leary & Diebels and Elkins-Brown et al., Chapters 4 and 5 in this volume). These basic constructs – automaticity and self – are central to most social psychological theories or models, and are crucial to understanding real life human behaviour.

Mindfulness and automatic versus controlled responding

The brain's capacity to regulate behaviour automatically and unconsciously is highly adaptive. Habitual and automatic response patterns can be extremely powerful in guiding us through life in a relatively effortless manner, allowing us to respond accurately and without much deliberation to the social and non-social environment (e.g. Custers & Aarts, 2010). At the same time, however, habitual and *mindless* responding may be at the root of various problems and challenges an individual may encounter in life. As discussed by Barsalou (Chapter 3 in this volume), life-long conditioned responses often remain unattended and outside of conscious awareness, while such responses may not necessarily be most effective in terms of increasing one's own well-being, or the well-being of relationships with others.

Typically, psychological theories assume that an automatically triggered behavioural response will be enacted. However, theorizing and research in mindfulness shows this link can be broken if attention is directed purposefully at the behavioural impulses themselves. Indeed, one of the central ideas of mindfulness is that it increases awareness of impulses, and while accepting these experiences as being merely transient mental events, an individual is able to prevent automatically acting on them, and can reconsider how to respond most effectively to his or her environment. In other words, mindfulness points to the potential for controlled processes to regulate automatic processes in novel ways – not by focusing on the *content* of thought, but by directing attention to their *nature* as mere mental events.

The chapters in this volume offer several examples of how mindfulness can reduce automatic responding and thus affect daily life outcomes. Papies (Chapter 7 in this volume) provides an overview of research suggesting that mindfulness can affect health-relevant behaviour, including healthy eating, smoking, and alcohol use. To explain such findings, she discusses how mindfulness promotes the monitoring of automatic impulses and cravings that often play a critical role in unhealthy behaviour. Becoming consciously aware of such impulses is a first prerequisite to reduce the otherwise automatic link between impulse and behavioural response (e.g. *mindlessly* lighting a cigarette when the impulse arises; *mindlessly* emptying a bag of potato chips in a habitual snacking situation). Importantly, however, a second prerequisite for not reacting to the impulse is to observe it from *a non-judgemental and decentered perspective*, which often allows the impulse to dissipate before it turns into actual behaviour.

Karremans and Kappen (Chapter 8 in this volume) discuss how a similar process may occur in the context of close relationships. Again, smooth interactions between partners may be guided by habitual responses, but certain habitual patterns may be the cause of relationship trouble. For example, as major social-psychological theories in relationship science recognize (e.g. interdependence theory; Rusbult & Van Lange, 1996), automatic tendencies to reciprocate a partner's negative behaviour can result in downward spirals of negativity, and often are at the heart of relationship decline. The ability to take a mindful and decentered perspective – paying close *attention* to feelings and action tendencies that arise in the present moment – should weaken the otherwise automatic association between impulses and outward behaviour toward the partner. More generally, although the role of attention to experiences that gives rise to experiential awareness has received little theoretical or empirical attention in relationship science, it may be an essential part of explaining the difference between ill- and well-functioning relationships.

Berry and Brown (Chapter 11 in this volume) discuss research indicating that mindfulness can positively affect intergroup prosociality by a similar process of de-automatizing. As the authors note, awareness of prejudiced responses is a crucial first step to attenuate the expression of prejudiced responses. Theory and research in the domain of prejudice and stereotyping clearly recognize the role of a *lack* of awareness of the activation of prejudiced feelings and impulses, or stereotypes, and of how this activation then automatically affects behaviour. Mindfulness may increase the ability to become aware of prejudiced feelings and impulses or the activation of a stereotype, allowing the mindful observer to "let it pass without reacting to it or acting on it" (p. 438; see Cox, Abramson, Devine, & Hollon, 2012). Thus, together, these examples illustrate how mindfulness and its intrinsic attention-related processes may weaken the automatic impulse-behaviour link and as such benefit individual, interpersonal, and intergroup outcomes.

Another way in which mindfulness may affect individual and interpersonal outcomes is its inverse relationship with mind-wandering (Mrazek, Smallwood, & Schooler, 2012). As most people probably have experienced, the mind has a strong and natural tendency to wander during whatever activity one engages in, which sometimes may hinder task-performance. Research indicates that mindfulness training is associated with noticing mind-wandering at earlier stages, allowing one to bring back attention to the task at hand (Mrazek et al., 2013). Mrazek and colleagues (Chapter 10 in this volume) discuss how the training of mindfulness in schools may increase sustained attention and hence improve academic achievement. These findings suggest that mindfulness can break the automaticity of task-unrelated cues leading to distraction and mind-wandering, with potential long-term benefits.

Health behaviour, close relationships, prejudice, and academic achievement are only a few examples of areas where mindfulness may have important consequences by affecting the interplay between automaticity and controlled processes. As future research should explore further, mindfulness may play a similar role in various other areas of social psychology where automaticity and controlled processing play prominent roles, such as attitude formation and change, social influence, cooperation and competition, impression formation, attribution processes, justice, social comparison, economic decision-making, and so on.

Mindfulness and self-related processes

As much as social psychology is concerned with the interplay of automatic and controlled processing, it is concerned with self-related processes. Constructs like self-esteem, self-construal, self-verification, self-enhancement, self-affirmation, self-perception, self-knowledge, and self-identity are topics that have been examined extensively in social psychology. This illustrates the emphasis in (Western) social psychological science on the self, and perhaps reflects a focus on the self in Western individualistic cultures more generally.

Leary and Diebels (Chapter 4 in this volume; see also Barsalou, Chapter 3 in this volume) argue that a change in how self-relevant information is processed may be at the core of many effects of mindfulness. Typically, people identify strongly with their experiences. Thoughts, sensations, and emotions are experienced as an integral part of the self (Bernstein et al., 2015), and produce a state that could be described as *subjective realism,* as the content of one's thoughts is experienced as reality (see Lebois et al., 2015; Papies, Pronk, Keesman, & Barsalou, 2015). While this may facilitate effective situated action (e.g. Barsalou, 2002), and support the construction of a coherent account of one's 'self' (Farb et al., 2007), this tendency is also associated with stress, rumination, and problematic cravings (e.g. Kross, Ayduk, & Mischel, 2005; Lebois et al., 2016).

In contrast, the decentered perspective that mindfulness entails facilitates a less immersed observing of the content of consciousness (see Hölzel et al., 2011, for an extensive discussion). For example, rather than being absorbed in distress, anger, or guilt, one observes these emotions as they arise and pass. The thoughts about one's self as a stable and 'real' construct can be observed from that perspective, too, which may decrease one's attachment to the static sense of self, or even lead to seeing it as an illusion (see Hölzel et al., 2011). As noted by Leary and Diebels (p. 53, in this volume), "mindfulness does not eliminate self-awareness or make people 'self-less'. Rather, it changes the amount and nature of self-attention and self-thought to be less self-focused and self-interested than it typically is."

Again, this should have important implications for various domains of social-psychological theory and research. Mindfulness may reduce self-defensive responding across various situations. For example, both prejudice, stereotyping, and interpersonal aggression have been argued to result at least partly from defending the self as part of an in-group and the desire to uphold a favourable view of the self, especially when provoked (e.g. Baumeister, Smart, & Boden, 1996; Tajfel, 1981; see Berry & Brown, Chapter 11 in this volume). Hence, by promoting a decentered perspective toward one's self-concept and one's experiences, mindfulness may reduce prejudice and less interpersonal aggression. Similar effects may be observed in other areas where self-defensive mechanisms play a central role, as suggested by a number of prominent theories in social psychology (e.g. self-affirmation theory, cognitive dissonance theory, terror management theory, and social identity theory).

Through a similar process, the less self-focused, decentered mode that is associated with mindfulness provides more opportunities for taking the perspective of others. Berry and Brown (Chapter 11 in this volume) describe how this process may foster intergroup prosociality. Condon (Chapter 9 this volume) reviews some initial research findings indicating that mindfulness indeed can promote compassion and prosocial behaviour in an interpersonal context. More generally, research suggests that both trait mindfulness and mindfulness training are positively associated with perspective taking and empathy (Birnie et al., 2010). Possibly, these findings can be explained in terms of less self-focus (or, as Leary and Giebels refer to, in terms of a "hypo-egoic mindset").

In sum, the research discussed so far suggests that changing attentional and self-related processes is a central effect of mindfulness, and engaging with mindfulness research may therefore provide useful insights for research in social psychology.

Implications for applications of social psychology

In addition to these theoretical and empirical contributions to modern social psychology, mindfulness may be of relevance to social psychologists because of the potential it offers for intervention tools that can fundamentally alter people's daily life experiences. This is particularly relevant as mindfulness-based interventions rely on the innate abilities of attention regulation and of taking a meta-cognitive perspective on one's own experiences, which are available to any human mind and can be tapped in a variety of ways. Indeed, the process of non-judgemental observation is not a skill that can be acquired through mindfulness training and meditation only, but is naturally available in human beings. Using attention skills, people have the unique ability to observe the content of consciousness, introspect, and adopt a meta-cognitive perspective on their experiences. While there seem to be considerable pre-existing individual differences (Brown & Ryan, 2003; see also Alberts, Chapter 2 in this volume), both attention regulation and meta-cognitive insight can be trained and cultivated further.

When developing interventions in the domains of health, relationship behaviour, workplace behaviour, stereotyping, intergroup contact, or others, social psychologists can capitalize on these existing abilities. The chapters in this volume provide numerous examples of how even brief or low-dose interventions enhance mindfulness skills enough to show meaningful behavioural effects. At the same time, the crucial mechanisms underlying mindfulness effects are not exclusive to meditation and mindfulness-based interventions. As a result, even interventions that are not explicitly 'mindfulness' can lead to benefits of improved attention regulation or a changed meta-cognitive perspective on one's experiences, and to associated effects on cognition and behaviour (for examples, see Kross, 2009; Luciano et al., 2011). Thus, in addition to contributing to theory in social psychology, research on mindfulness can further inform applications to target critical societal issues.

The value of social psychology for mindfulness research and practice

While knowledge about the psychological and neurophysiological effects of mindfulness has expanded rapidly, considerable work remains to be done to fully understand *how* and *when* mindfulness works. For example, a basic social-psychological principle is that an individual's emotional and behavioural responses to others, and towards oneself, result from the individual's construal of the situation. How mindfulness may affect such construal processes is largely unexplored territory, but we suggest that such research should be informed by existing social psychological theories. More generally, social psychology is strongly concerned with fine-grained analyses of the specific psychological mechanisms that underlie our experiences and behaviour. This volume presents various examples of how this may benefit mindfulness research. While the link between mindfulness and self-control has repeatedly been demonstrated, Elkins-Brown, Teper, and Inzlicht (Chapter 5 this volume) discuss in detail *how* mindfulness actually may improve self-control. In short, they argue that non-judgemental interoceptive awareness promotes the monitoring of conflict-related affect, which in turn should facilitate self-control. Similarly, based on a classic social-psychological model of emotion regulation (Gross, 1998), Slutsky, Rahl, Lindsay, and Creswell (Chapter 6 in this volume) discuss how mindfulness may impact emotion regulation at various stages of the model. Further, as discussed earlier, the chapters by Leary and Diebels and by Barsalou (Chapters 4 and 3 in this volume) describe how mindfulness effects can be better understood through closely analyzing self-related and attention-related processes. Thus, the process-focus that characterizes social psychological research can bring important insights to the field of mindfulness.

Moreover, social psychologists have a strong tradition of testing their theories experimentally. So far, a large number of studies in the mindfulness literature have examined the relationship between (often trait) mindfulness and other variables in correlational designs, making it impossible to draw conclusions about causality. Stronger evidence in support of mindfulness effects is derived from randomized controlled trials in clinical psychology, in which the effect of mindfulness training is contrasted with an active control condition (see Creswell, in press). However, based on such studies, it is difficult to deduce what specific elements of the training are responsible for the effect. As we will discuss in more detail, experimental paradigms in social psychology can advance the field by zooming in on the specific factors that drive mindfulness effects. In addition, social psychological research has produced various research tools to assess unconscious and implicit processes (see Gawronski & De Houwer, 2014) that constitute an important and emerging addition to current research findings in the field of mindfulness, which have traditionally been based mainly on explicit self-report measures.

In addition to its potential for theoretical and methodological advancement in basic mindfulness research, a social-psychological perspective on mindfulness may help trainers and practitioners to better understand the full potential of mindfulness for daily life. Whereas the emphasis of mindfulness-based interventions so far typically is on stress reduction and individual well-being, training programs could benefit from more specific social-psychological knowledge regarding how effects of mindfulness may surface in various aspects of daily life. This is especially important given that research syntheses suggest that the effects of relatively short mindfulness-based interventions may be domain-specific, rather than generalizing across domains of life where mindfulness effects might be seen as desirable (see Papies, Chapter 7 this volume).

Conclusion and future challenges

So, why should social psychologists care about mindfulness? As noted, classic social psychology (and psychology more broadly) is mostly concerned with the specific contents of human cognition, emotion, and behaviour, and how these affect our lives and social fabric. Mindfulness, in contrast, focuses on whether and how people observe and relate to their experiences that arise in consciousness, irrespective of their specific content. This is not something 'invented' by mindfulness practitioners and scholars. Rather, people vary naturally from moment to moment, and from situation to situation, in their tendency to be fully immersed in their experiences, or to observe them from a more detached perspective. The mindfulness literature provides strong theoretical and methodological guidance for understanding each of these processing modes, their consequences, and how people can switch between them – issues that we suggest may have been largely overlooked by social psychological theories so far. Hence, we strongly believe that social psychology as a field could benefit from mindfulness research, in order to advance fundamental knowledge and theory about human experiences and behaviour, and because mindfulness as an intervention tool offers potentially powerful ways to improve people's daily lives.

The current volume provides an overview of mindfulness research that may illustrate this. We hope that recent developments in this area are just the beginning of much more to come, and particularly, our hope is that insights from mindfulness research will find a more central place in social psychology. After the first wave (i.e. "Does it work?"), and the second wave of mindfulness research (i.e. "How does it work?"), social psychologists could contribute greatly to a third wave of research that examines the broader applications of mindfulness in daily life, going beyond the question of whether mindfulness reduces stress and improves well-being.

Before closing, however, we wish to highlight some challenges that may require additional attention as the field moves forward. First, reading this chapter and reading this entire volume, one could be led to believe that mindfulness is a panacea that will solve all problems in one's personal life, and in society at large. Most likely, it's not. First of all, it is not clear for whom, and under which circumstances, mindfulness may be particularly beneficial, and whether, for example, its benefits depend on factors such as one's level of education, cultural background, or the expectancy that one will benefit from the training. Also, as we have discussed elsewhere (Karremans, Schellekens, & Kappen, 2015), it is not yet known whether mindfulness perhaps undermines *functional* automaticity in everyday life. If mindfulness becomes a habitual way of responding to situations, is there less leeway for otherwise beneficial automatic processes? Very little research has addressed questions about the boundaries of mindfulness effects, and attempts to study its potential harmful or negative effects are nearly absent (for an exception, see for example Wilson et al., 2015).

Another current challenge relates to the fact that the strong ethical context that plays a major role in contemplative practice in traditional Buddhism – focusing on the development of 'right' mindfulness, wisdom, and the cessation of suffering – is much less explicit in contemporary mindfulness, which often focuses more on short-term, symptomatic relief (see Condon, Chapter 9 in this volume; Monteiro, Musten, & Compson, 2015). This has triggered significant controversy and points to the need for continuing dialogue between scientists studying mindfulness and traditional mindfulness communities and philosophers (e.g. Dunne, 2015; Monteiro et al., 2015). The strong integration of ethical principles of behaviour into mindfulness-based interventions is of particular relevance to social psychologists, as this may ultimately benefit interpersonal and intergroup relationships. A related issue that will require consideration by researchers is the increased attention to so-called varieties of contemplative experience. These can include adverse effects of meditation practice that have been reported by meditation practitioners, particularly after intense practice of techniques that are also often used in mindfulness-based interventions, albeit less intensely (Crouch, 2013; Kornfield, 1979). Again, although systematic research into these phenomena is still only beginning to emerge, this is an important caveat for those who wish to employ mindfulness interventions, particularly if this happens on a wider scale and without close supervision by experienced teachers.

A further challenge concerns the methods for studying mindfulness. Alberts (Chapter 2 this volume) provides an overview of existing lab- and non-lab methods to investigate mindfulness effects, discussing both their strengths and pitfalls. For example, contrasting the effects of a mindfulness training, meditation, or brief mindfulness induction with a control condition generally involves many potential confounds (e.g. group processes in training, relaxation as a result of a mindfulness exercise, expectancies). Hence, one particular challenge concerns the issue of what constitutes a proper control condition. Moreover, while brief mindfulness inductions are increasingly used by psychological scientists, mindfulness researchers and practitioners have been critical about the validity of such brief inductions, especially when using research participants with no previous mindfulness experience. Similarly, self-report measures of mindfulness have been criticized for a variety of measurement problems (Grossman & Van Dam, 2011). Thus, while social psychological experimental methods may offer novel ways to study mindfulness, these methods should be used with an awareness of such potential problems.

As with any maturing field, it will take effort to overcome such challenges, and it will take time to get a complete and nuanced picture of the workings and correlates of the rich and multifaceted concept of mindfulness. It is our hope that the present volume will contribute to this process.

Acknowledgement

We would like to thank Madelijn Strick, Gesa Kappen, and Martijn de Lange for helpful comments on an earlier version of this chapter.

Note

1 There is quite some debate about the definition of mindfulness in the context of Buddhist traditions. Some argue that the contemporary, scientific use of the term *mindfulness* has only some overlap with Buddhist conceptions of the term; some have argued that the secular conceptualization of mindfulness has stripped down the full meaning and potential of mindfulness, including its ethical implications (for discussions, see for example Dunne, 2015; Monteiro et al., 2015). Although we agree that a more profound integration of Buddhist and Western psychology is valuable and perhaps even necessary, this debate is beyond the scope of the present volume. The chapters in this book essentially follow the definition of mindfulness as described in this introduction chapter.

References

Baer, R.A. (Ed.). (2015). *Mindfulness-based treatment approaches: Clinician's guide to evidence base and applications.* Academic Press.

Barsalou, L.W. (2002). Being there conceptually: Simulating categories in preparation for situated action. In N. Stein, P. Bauer, & M. Rabinowita (Eds.) *Representation, memory, and development: Essays in honor of Jean Mandler,* 1–15. Mahwah, NJ: Lawrence Erlbaum.

Baumeister, R. F., Smart, L., & Boden, J. M. (1996). Relation of threatened egotism to violence and aggression: The dark side of high self-esteem. *Psychological Review, 103*(1), 5.

Bernstein, A., Hadash, Y., Lichtash, Y., Tanay, G., Shepherd, K., & Fresco, D. M. (2015). Decentering and related constructs: A critical review and metacognitive processes model. *Perspectives on Psychological Science, 10*(5), 599–617.

Birnie, K., Speca, M., & Carlson, L. E. (2010). Exploring self-compassion and empathy in the context of mindfulness-based stress reduction (MBSR). *Stress and Health, 26*(5), 359–371.

Bishop, S. R., Lau, M., Shapiro, S., Carlson, L., Anderson, N. D., Carmody, J., . . . Devins, G. (2004). Mindfulness: A proposed operational definition. *Clinical Psychology: Science and Practice, 11*(3), 230–241.

Brown, K.W., & Ryan, R. M. (2003). The benefits of being present: Mindfulness and its role in psychological well-being. *Journal of Personality and Social Psychology, 84*(4), 822.

Chambers, R., Lo, B. C.Y., & Allen, N. B. (2008). The impact of intensive mindfulness training on attentional control, cognitive style, and affect. *Cognitive Therapy and Research, 32*(3), 303–322.

Chen, M., & Bargh, J. A. (1999). Consequences of automatic evaluation: Immediate behavioral predispositions to approach or avoid the stimulus. *Personality and Social Psychology Bulletin, 25*(2), 215–224.

Cox, W.T., Abramson, L.Y., Devine, P. G., & Hollon, S. D. (2012). Stereotypes, prejudice, and depression: The integrated perspective. *Perspectives on Psychological Science, 7*(5), 427–449.

Creswell, J.D. (in press). Mindfulness interventions. *Annual Review of Psychology.*

Crouch, R. (2013, July 23). The refugees of mindfulness: Rethinking psychology's experiment with meditation. Retrieved from https://alohadharma.com/2013/07/23/the-refugees-of-mindfulness-rethinking-psychologys-experiment-with-meditation/

Custers, R., & Aarts, H. (2010). The unconscious will: How the pursuit of goals operates outside of conscious awareness. *Science, 329*(5987), 47–50.

Davidson, R. J., Kabat-Zinn, J., Schumacher, J., Rosenkranz, M., Muller, D., Santorelli, S. F., ... Sheridan, J. F. (2003). Alterations in brain and immune function produced by mindfulness meditation. *Psychosomatic medicine, 65*(4), 564–570.

Dunne, J. D. (2015). Buddhist styles of mindfulness: A heuristic approach. In B. D. Ostafin, M. D. Robinson, & B. P. Meier (Eds.), *Mindfulness and Self-regulation* (pp. 251–270). New York: Springer.

Epstein, M. (2008). *Psychotherapy without the self: A Buddhist perspective.* New Haven, CT: Yale University Press.

Farb, N. A. S., Segal, Z. V., Mayberg, H., Bean, J., McKeon, D., Fatima, Z., & Anderson, A. K. (2007). Attending to the present: Mindfulness meditation reveals distinct neural modes of self-reference. *Social Cognitive and Affective Neuroscience, 2*(4), 313–322.

Gawronski, B., & De Houwer, J. (2014). Implicit measures in social and personality psychology. In H. T. Reis & C. M. Judd (Eds.), *Handbook of research methods in social and personality psychology* (2nd ed.; pp. 283–310). New York: Cambridge University Press.

Goldin, P. R., & Gross, J. J. (2010). Effects of mindfulness-based stress reduction (MBSR) on emotion regulation in social anxiety disorder. *Emotion, 10*(1), 83–91.

Greenwald, A. G., & Banaji, M. R. (1995). Implicit social cognition: Attitudes, self-esteem, and stereotypes. *Psychological Review, 102*(1), 4.

Gross, J. J. (1998). The emerging field of emotion regulation: An integrative review. *Review of General Psychology, 2*(3), 271–299.

Gross, J. J., & John, O. P. (2003). Individual differences in two emotion regulation processes: Implications for affect, relationships, and well-being. *Journal of Personality and Social Psychology, 85*(2), 348.

Grossman, P., & Van Dam, N. T. (2011). Mindfulness, by any other name. . .: Trials and tribulations of sati in Western psychology and science. *Contemporary Buddhism, 12*(1), 219–239.

Herring, D. R., White, K. R., Jabeen, L. N., Hinojos, M., Terrazas, G., Reyes, S. M., ... Crites, S. L., Jr. (2013). On the automatic activation of attitudes: A quarter century of evaluative priming research. *Psychological Bulletin*, No Pagination Specified.

Hölzel, B. K., Lazar, S. W., Gard, T., Schuman-Olivier, Z., Vago, D. R., & Ott, U. (2011). How does mindfulness meditation work? Proposing mechanisms of action from a conceptual and neural perspective. *Perspectives on Psychological Science, 6*(6), 537–559.

Kabat-Zinn, J. (1982). An outpatient program in behavioral medicine for chronic pain patients based on the practice of mindfulness meditation: Theoretical considerations and preliminary results. *General Hospital Psychiatry, 4*(1), 33–47.

Kabat-Zinn, J. (1990). *Full catastrophe living: Using the wisdom of your body and mind to face stress, pain and illness.* New York: Delacorte.

Kabat-Zinn, J. (1994). *Wherever you go, there you are.* New York: Hyperion Books.

Kabat-Zinn, J., Lipworth, L., & Burney, R. (1985). The clinical use of mindfulness meditation for the self-regulation of chronic pain. *Journal of Behavioral Medicine, 8*(2), 163–190.

Karremans, J. C., Schellekens, M. P., & Kappen, G. (2015). Bridging the sciences of mindfulness and romantic relationships: A theoretical model and research agenda. *Personality and Social Psychology Review, 21,* 29–49. doi:1088868315615450.

Killingsworth, M. A., & Gilbert, D. T. (2010). A wandering mind is an unhappy mind. *Science, 330*(6006), 932–932.

Kornfield, J. (1979). Intensive insight meditation: A phenomenological study. *The Journal of Transpersonal Psychology, 11*(1), 41.

Kross, E. (2009). When the self becomes other. *Annals of the New York Academy of Sciences, 1167,* 35–40.

Kross, E., Ayduk, O., & Mischel, W. (2005). When asking "Why" does not hurt. Distinguishing rumination from reflective processing of negative emotions. *Psychological Science, 16*(9), 709–715.

Langer, E. J. (1989). *Mindfulness.* Reading, MA: Addison-Wesley/Addison Wesley Longman.

Lebois, L. A. M., Hertzog, C., Slavich, G. M., Barrett, L. F., & Barsalou, L. W. (2016). Establishing the situated features associated with perceived stress. *Acta Psychologica, 169,* 119–132.

Lebois, L. A. M., Papies, E. K., Gopinath, K., Cabanban, R., Quigley, K. S., Krishnamurthy, V., . . . Barsalou, L. W. (2015). A shift in perspective: Decentering through mindful attention to imagined stressful events. *Neuropsychologia, 75,* 505–524.

Luciano, C., Ruiz, F. J., Vizcaíno Torres, R. M., Sánchez Martín, V., Gutiérrez Martínez, O., López, J. C. (2011). A relational frame analysis of defusion in acceptance and commitment therapy: A preliminary and quasi-experimental study with at-risk adolescents. *International Journal of Psychology and Psychological Therapy, 11,* 165–182.

Miller, J. J., Fletcher, K., & Kabat-Zinn, J. (1995). Three-year follow-up and clinical implications of a mindfulness meditation-based stress reduction intervention in the treatment of anxiety disorders. *General Hospital Psychiatry, 17*(3), 192–200.

Monteiro, L. M., Musten, R. F., & Compson, J. (2015). Traditional and contemporary mindfulness: Finding the middle path in the tangle of concerns. *Mindfulness, 6*(1), 1–13.

Mrazek, M. D., Franklin, M. S., Phillips, D. T., Baird, B., & Schooler, J. W. (2013). Mindfulness training improves working memory capacity and GRE performance while reducing mind wandering. *Psychological Science, 24,* 776–781. doi:0956797612459659

Mrazek, M. D., Smallwood, J., & Schooler, J. W. (2012). Mindfulness and mind-wandering: Finding convergence through opposing constructs. *Emotion, 12*(3), 442.

Papies, E. K., Pronk, T. M., Keesman, M., & Barsalou, L. W. (2015). The benefits of simply observing: Mindful attention modulates the link between motivation and behavior. *Journal of Personality and Social Psychology, 108*(1), 148–170.

Rusbult, C. E., & Van Lange, P. A. M. (1996). Interdependence processes. In E. T. Higgins & A. W. Kruglanski (Eds.), *Social psychology: Handbook of basic principles* (pp. 564–596). New York: Guilford Press.

Snyder, M. (1974). Self-monitoring of expressive behavior. *Journal of Personality and Social Psychology, 30*(4), 526.

Tajfel, H. (1981). *Human groups and social categories: Studies in social psychology.* CUP Archive.

Teasdale, J. D., Segal, Z., & Williams, J. M. G. (1995). How does cognitive therapy prevent depressive relapse and why should attentional control (mindfulness) training help? *Behaviour Research and Therapy, 33*(1), 25–39.

Teper, R., Segal, Z. V., & Inzlicht, M. (2013). Inside the mindful mind: How mindfulness enhances emotion regulation through improvements in executive control. *Current Directions in Psychological Science, 22*(6), 449–454.

Wicklund, R. A. (1975). Objective self-awareness. *Advances in Experimental Social Psychology, 8,* 233–275.

Williams, J. M. G., & Kabat-Zinn, J. (2013). *Mindfulness: Diverse perspectives on its meaning, origins and applications.* New York: Routledge.

Wilson, B. M., Mickes, L., Stolarz-Fantino, S., Evrard, M., & Fantino, E. (2015). Increased false-memory susceptibility after mindfulness meditation. *Psychological Science, 26*(10), 1567–1573.

Wyer, R. S. (2014). *The automaticity of everyday life: Advances in social cognition* (Vol. 10). New York: Psychology Press.

Zeidan, F., Martucci, K. T., Kraft, R. A., Gordon, N. S., McHaffie, J. G., & Coghill, R. C. (2011). Brain mechanisms supporting the modulation of pain by mindfulness meditation. *The Journal of Neuroscience, 31*(14), 5540–5548.

2

STUDYING MINDFULNESS WITH DIFFERENT METHODS

Hugo J.E.M. Alberts

Mindfulness, the "awareness of present experience with acceptance" (Germer, 2005), has received considerable scholarly attention. Over the last decade, psychological research on mindfulness has increased strongly. Whereas initial studies mainly concerned clinical topics and intrapersonal processes, later research began to address mindfulness in other areas as well, including the social domain. Although mindfulness has only recently begun to attain a more pronounced position in the field of social psychology, addressing the impact of self-awareness from an intrapersonal perspective is certainly not new. In the history of social psychology, many studies have addressed the human ability to become an object of one's own consciousness (see for instance Duval & Wicklund, 1972) and revealed that awareness of the self, including reflecting or thinking about the self, can strongly influence interaction with the social environment (see also Leary & Diebels, Chapter 4 in this volume).

In this light, it is perhaps no surprise that higher levels of mindfulness have consistently been found to influence interaction with the social environment. For instance, increased mindfulness has been related to more prosocial behaviour (Flook, Goldberg, Pinger, & Davidson, 2015), and more positive interpersonal interactions (Dekeyser et al., 2008; see also Karremans & Kappen, Chapter 8 in this volume; Leary & Diebels, Chapter 4 in this volume). In fact, Van Doesum and colleagues (2013) coined the term "social mindfulness" to describe the human ability to "safeguard other people's control over their own behavioural options in situations of interdependence (p. 86)".

The findings described earlier suggest that investigating the relationship between mindfulness and social psychology may enhance understanding of the processes underlying social interaction that promote well-being at a personal and interpersonal level. The present chapter aims to facilitate the development of research on mindfulness in the field of social psychology by providing a comprehensive overview of the different methods for studying mindfulness. In addition, both the advantages and limitations of the research methods will be critically examined. In this way, we hope to provide a useful tool for researchers to design studies that help to enrich our understanding of mindfulness and contribute to convergent evidence.

In the first part of this chapter, we focus on different ways to increase mindfulness, either by structurally training or temporarily inducing mindfulness. Next, we discuss different tools for assessing both state and trait mindfulness, and discuss their strengths and weaknesses. Finally, we consider different factors that are important to take into consideration when designing mindfulness experiments.

Increasing mindfulness

The growth in mindfulness research has been accompanied by the development of a great diversity of methods to increase mindfulness, both in and outside the lab. In this section we distinguish between long-term interventions, low-dose interventions and experimentally induced mindfulness.

Long-term interventions

Long-term mindfulness interventions are typically employed in the field of clinical psychology. Most of these interventions involve 8 weeks of training. For instance, mindfulness-based stress reduction (MBSR: Kabat-Zinn, 1982) and mindfulness-based cognitive therapy (MBCT: Segal, Williams, & Teasdale, 2002) include eight weekly meetings and daily practice. Typically, the weekly sessions take 2 hours or more and consist of mindfulness practices (e.g. breath awareness or mindful yoga) and discussing the homework, exercises and experiences of the last week. In between meetings, participants are encouraged to conduct formal mindfulness practices at home on a daily basis for about 45 minutes.

The rationale behind this high level of practice is that mindfulness cannot be regarded as a quick solution to problems. Many problems, like addiction, depression or out-group aggression involve strong habitual and cognitive patterns that are unlikely to be altered by employing a one-time mindfulness meditation (see also Barsalou, Chapter 3 in this volume). Long-term mindfulness interventions address these problems in a structural and profound way, thereby increasing the likelihood of achieving observable and sustainable effects. In addition, when aiming to bridge the gap between research and (clinical) practice, the protocol that is tested in long-term interventions can often be used directly in the practical field.

Long-term interventions that employ regular group meetings may provide an interesting context for studying the link between mindfulness and social psychology. So far, most studies addressing this link have focused on the identification of social outcomes that are affected by mindfulness. However, preliminary evidence suggests that the social context can also influence the development of mindfulness. Individuals who grow up in an environment that is characterized by a reliably available, sensitive and responsive interaction with caregivers are likely to develop higher levels of mindfulness as adults (Shaver, Lavy, Saron, & Mikulincer, 2007).

In a similar way, group sessions may facilitate the development of mindfulness through the creation of a safe social environment that promotes beneficial intra- and interpersonal processes. Addressing social processes that enhance or reduce mindfulness may shed more light on the social foundations of mindfulness.

Low-dose interventions

While most clinical mindfulness programs have adopted the 8-week framework described earlier, the expansion of mindfulness in non-clinical fields has led to the development of interventions characterized by a different duration. Examples of variations in terms of duration include four 50-minute sessions within a 3-week period (Jennings & Jennings, 2013), three weekly 45-min sessions of meditation exercises (Call, Miron, & Orcutt, 2013), and four 45-min sessions four times a week for 2 week (Mrazek et al., 2013). While the MBSR program requires participants to commit to about 45 minutes of daily mindfulness practice, low-dose interventions typically require less time of home practice, for instance 10 minutes (Mrazek et al., 2013) or even no home practice at all (Call, Miron, & Orcutt, 2013; Jennings & Jennings, 2013).

Long-term interventions typically require a high level of time investment, from participants as well as trainers. Low-dose interventions offer the possibility to study the effects of repeated mindfulness practice in a more time (and cost) effective way. Research findings confirm that structural, pronounced changes can be accomplished by using low-dose interventions. For instance, even after 4 weeks of mindfulness training, structural changes in the brain have been observed (for an overview, see Tang, Hölzel, & Posner, 2015), and undertaking 30 mins of daily mindfulness meditation over a 3-week period has been found to significantly increase cognitive empathy (Keefe, 1979).

On the negative side, studying mindfulness using longer-term interventions, including low-dose interventions, provides little insight in the exact working mechanisms and effectiveness of the different methods used in the intervention. In fact, the selection of methods that have been employed in longer-term, low-dose interventions differs greatly among studies. While some interventions use breathing meditations only, others include additional practices, like body-scan and 3-minute coping (Kabat-Zinn, 1982, 1990). Moreover, the number of group meetings and the extent to which participants received psycho-education also differs greatly among studied interventions. As a result, it is not only difficult to compare different programs, it also remains unclear which elements of an intervention are responsible or necessary for results, and how these elements interact with each other. One way to enhance comparability of mindfulness interventions is by using standardized protocols.

Experimentally induced mindfulness

In most laboratory studies, participants are instructed to apply mindfulness exercises for a brief period of time. Typically, participants are exposed to a guided meditation in the form of a pre-recorded instruction. For example, after a 5-minute mindfulness meditation, a study by Tan, Lo, and Macrae (2014) revealed that participants' mental state attribution and empathic concern was enhanced as compared to a control group, who did not engage in mindfulness meditation.

Over the past years, a diverse range of manipulations to experimentally induce a state of mindfulness have been developed. Examples include performing a "raisin-eating" task (Kabat-Zinn, 1990; Ramsey & Jones, 2015), using mindful self-focus statements on cards (Kuehner, Huffziger, & Liebsch, 2009) and applying mindfulness instructions while watching an emotional video (Alberts, Schneider, & Martijn, 2012).

Conducting research under controlled experimental settings can enhance understanding on the working mechanisms of mindfulness. For instance, in a study by Lueke and Gibson (2014), exposure to a brief mindfulness meditation caused a decrease in implicit out-group bias. Analysis revealed that this decrease could partly be attributed to a reduction in the automatic activation of negative associations. These findings shed light on possible mechanisms by showing that automatic associations are reduced in a mindful state of awareness (see also Barsalou, Chapter 3 in this volume; Papies, Chapter 7 in this volume).

Assessing trait mindfulness

Trait or dispositional mindfulness can be defined as an individual's baseline or average level of mindfulness. It refers to an individual's capacity and "tendency to abide in mindful states over time" (Brown, Ryan, & Creswell, 2007, p. 218). In this section we review different ways to measure interpersonal differences in trait mindfulness, including their benefits and limitations.

Self-report measures

Studies addressing the development of self-report measures of trait mindfulness have shown that individuals differ in their natural levels of mindfulness. These interpersonal differences have been found to be predictive of a wide variety of psychological outcomes, both relating to intrapersonal and interpersonal processes.

For instance, high dispositional mindfulness is related to satisfaction with interpersonal relationships (Pepping, O'Donovan, Zimmer-Gembeck, & Hanisch, 2014) and forgiveness (Oman et al., 2008; see also Karremans & Kappen, Chapter 8 in this volume). During the past 15 years, a wide variety of mindfulness self-report measures have been developed, varying in scope and targeting different sets of mindfulness elements.

One of the most popular measures is the Mindful Attention Awareness Scale (MAAS, Brown & Ryan, 2003). The scale addresses the general tendency to be aware of and attentive to present-moment experiences in daily life. Respondents indicate to which extent they act on automatic pilot or pay attention to the present moment. Research found that the scale has good psychometric properties and shows strong positive relations with different measures of well-being and strong inverse relations with measures of physical symptoms (Brown & Ryan, 2003). Moreover, scores on the MAAS have been found to be associated with differential patterns of brain activity (e.g. Creswell, Way, Eisenberger, & Lieberman, 2007) and treatment outcomes (e.g. Michalak, Heidenreich, Meibert, & Schulte, 2008).

Despite the popularity of the MAAS, some researchers have argued that measuring mindfulness as a single-faceted construct fails to take into account the complexity of the construct. Consequently, several multifaceted mindfulness questionnaires have been designed. The Philadelphia Mindfulness Scale (PHLMS; Cardaciotto et al., 2008) addresses both present-moment awareness and acceptance. Respondents indicate how frequently a series of 20 experiences occurred during the past week. Another scale that addresses even a wider range of factors than the PHILMS is the Five Facet Mindfulness Questionnaire (FFMQ; Baer et al., 2006). This scale assesses five distinct mindfulness skills: observing phenomena mindfully, describing one's thoughts and feelings, acting with awareness, non-judging of inner experience and non-reactivity to inner experience. The scale has been found to be both reliable and valid (see for instance Bohlmeijer et al., 2011). In a similar vein, The Kentucky Inventory of Mindfulness Skills (KIMS; Baer, Smith, & Allen, 2004) addresses four components of mindfulness: observing, describing, acting with awareness and accepting without judgement. Other multifaceted scales that have been used to address trait mindfulness are The Child and Adolescent Mindfulness Measure (Greco, Baer, & Smith, 2011), and The Cognitive and Affective Mindfulness Scale (CAMS; Feldman et al., 2007), all addressing mindfulness based on a different conceptualization of the construct and targeting populations that differ in their experience with mindfulness.

Several authors have emphasized important concerns with self-reports of mindfulness (see for instance Grossman, 2008). First, the great variety of mindfulness questionnaires illustrates an absence of agreement in how to define the concept. Even among experts, consensus on the exact components and defining characteristics is currently lacking. For instance, while measures like the KIMS and FFMQ differentiate between five underlying factors, the MAAS assesses only one single factor. Consequently, objectively comparing results between studies that employed different mindfulness measures is problematic. Moreover, research findings suggest that correlations of trait mindfulness with other constructs seem to vary across scales (see for instance Schmertz, Anderson, & Robins, 2009).

Another critical issue related to mindfulness self-reports concerns the introspective skills that are required for accurately measuring the construct. Mindfulness can be described as a form of self-reflection and meta-awareness. Higher levels of mindfulness imply that one is better able to take the stance of an observer, allowing one to more objectively and accurately describe inner processes. Obviously, self-report measures rely heavily on self-reflection and introspection, suggesting that the meta-awareness that is cultivated through mindfulness may be an important pre-requisite for accurate measurement. From this perspective, measuring awareness by asking individuals how aware they are may yield results that are not always equally good reflections of the underlying construct.

Finally, after completing a mindfulness intervention, the concepts measured by the mindfulness questionnaires are easily recognizable for participants. This can be problematic, especially in combination with the possibility that the answers of participants who have invested a lot of time and effort into their practice may, at least partly, reflect wishing or believing that mindfulness qualities have developed (Grossman, 2008).

Meditation experience

Previous research has revealed a relationship between meditation experience and levels of mindfulness. For instance, in a study by Vinchurkar, Singh, and Visweswaraiah (2014), years of meditation practice were found to be significantly correlated with levels of trait mindfulness. Following this, a possible way to assess mindfulness levels and differentiate between low and high levels of mindfulness is to assess participants' prior experience with meditation. On the basis of daily practice and time spent in meditation retreats, a total amount of hours of meditation training can be estimated (see for instance Hölzel et al., 2008). In most studies, this assessment of trait mindfulness is used as a way to create control (no prior experience with meditation) versus experimental groups (a high level of mindfulness meditation experience).

Although meditation experience may seem a relatively objective indication of trait mindfulness, it must be recognized that meditation does not equal mindfulness. Irrespective of formal meditation experience, dispositional mindfulness levels appear to vary among the population (Brown & Ryan, 2003) and mindfulness can be practiced in many different ways other than (formal) meditation. In other words, although meditation experience may be perceived as a reliable predictor of trait mindfulness, the absence of meditation experience does not necessarily imply lower levels of mindfulness.

Assessing state mindfulness

In addition to trait mindfulness, mindfulness can also refer to state or quality of awareness (Brown & Ryan, 2003). In a mindful state, an individual is directing attention toward the present moment in an open and receptive way (Brown, Ryan, & Creswell, 2007). In this section we address different ways of assessing state mindfulness.

Self-report measures

State mindfulness can be measured with the Toronto Mindfulness Scale (TMS; Lau et al., 2006) and the state MAAS (Brown & Ryan, 2003). The TMS measures the extent to which participants were aware and accepting of their experiences during a previous meditation or other mindfulness exercise. Studies have revealed that brief mindfulness inductions can increase state levels of mindfulness, as reflected by higher scores on the TMS (see for instance Garland, Hanley, Farb, & Froeliger, 2013).

The state version of the MAAS aims to assess the current expression of a mindful state of mind, that is, a receptive state of mind characterized by a sensitive awareness of what is occurring in the present moment. While the state MAAS is often used as a single-time measurement of mindful awareness (e.g. during an experimental session), it has also been used to capture mindfulness over time. For instance, in a study by Hulsheger, Alberts, Feinholdt, and Lang (2012), experience sampling using the state MAAS was employed to measure daily levels of mindfulness over a period of five consecutive days.

Behavioural correlates

In order to quantify levels of mindfulness, previous studies have addressed the link between mindfulness and different behavioural markers that are assumed to reflect core components of the concept. For instance, focused attention, a core component of mindfulness, has been found to be enhanced after a brief mindfulness meditation as indicated by a reduction in mind-wandering during a Sustained Attention to Response Task (Mrazek, Smallwood, & Schooler, 2012). Moreover, in an experiment by Frewen and colleagues (2008), the process of focused attention was measured during meditation practice. Participants were exposed to a 15-minute meditation during which every 3 minutes a bell rang. When this bell rang, participants were instructed to raise their right hand if their attention was focused on their breathing, and raise their left hand if their attention had wandered to another activity (e.g. thinking). The total number of times a participant had been focused on his breathing was translated to a frequency score from 0 to 5, referred to by the authors as the "Meditation Breath Attention Score". Participants who scored higher on trait mindfulness were found to have higher scores on this measure.

Another component of mindfulness, reduced emotional reactivity, has also been found to be affected by brief mindfulness inductions. For instance, a study by Arch and Craske (2006) showed that participants who were exposed to a brief mindfulness meditation reported less negative emotional reactivity in response to affectively valenced slides compared to controls. In a similar vein, a study by Broderick (2005) revealed that a brief mindfulness meditation caused participants in the experimental condition to recover faster from a sad mood induction compared to a distraction condition. Decreased emotional reactivity has also been measured using biological markers, for instance sympathetic arousal (Carlson, Speca, Faris, & Patel, 2007; Ortner, Kilner, & Zelazo, 2007) and amygdala activity (Creswell, Way, Eisenberger, & Lieberman, 2007; Taylor et al., 2011).

It is important to bear in mind that attempts to measure mindfulness by addressing one or few (behavioural) correlates imply a reduction of the concept. As stated previously, mindfulness can be perceived as a multifaceted construct that is unlikely to be fully captured by addressing only one or few of its components. Nevertheless, finding novel and relatively objective ways to measure the construct, albeit in a fragmented way, will not only contribute to convergent evidence but will also enhance our understanding of the underlying working mechanisms.

Practical advice

In this final section we focus on different factors that are important to consider when designing experiments and conducting research on mindfulness.

Designing control conditions

From a methodological perspective, the comparability of conditions is a core factor to consider when assigning participants to different groups. When considering mindfulness research, this means that instructions and interventions that are used to enhance mindfulness and the control interventions used, both in lab studies and (long-term) field studies, should be comparable in terms of style and length. However, given the complex and multifaceted nature of the construct, this can be a challenging task.

Many studies have used passive control groups: control conditions in which there are no instructions or interventions employed at all. For instance, in a lab study by Alberts and Thewissen (2011), participants in the experimental group were exposed to a brief mindfulness meditation, while participants in the control group skipped the meditation and started with the subsequent task immediately. In a similar vein, long-term and low-dose mindfulness interventions are often compared to a waiting-list control group who does not receive any kind of intervention or treatment (see for instance Chambers, Chuen Yee Lo, & Allen, 2008).

Among studies that employed active control groups, many differences can be observed. Some studies have used control conditions that were solely matched in terms of (assumed) task intensity and duration. For instance, in a study by Ramsey and Jones (2015), participants in the mindfulness condition performed a "raisin-eating" task while participants in the control condition engaged in a filler activity for the same duration; a typing task in which participants were asked to simply copy a passage of text by typing it verbatim. The rationale behind this task was that its neutral nature is unlikely to affect participants' mindfulness levels. Other studies have attempted to design control conditions that were predominantly matched in terms of delivery characteristics. In a study by Erisman and Roemer (2010), a brief mindfulness meditation was compared to a control group who was exposed to "neutral" educational information. When using pre-recorded audio instructions, as in this study, an advantage is that the similarity between the two conditions can easily be matched in terms of duration, tone of voice and number of words used. Long-term and low-dose studies using active control groups have also shown that it is possible to create comparable conditions, often in terms of duration, delivery mode and frequency. A elegant demonstration comes from Allen and colleagues (2012). In their study, a 6-week longitudinal trial of mindfulness training was compared to a reading group, who also met once per week, in the same building, for a similar duration of instruction every week. Additionally, participants received a CD with either 20 minutes of guided meditation instruction or 20-minute excerpts from a book. All participants completed 20 minutes of home practice per day.

An important factor that influences appropriate active control group selection is the component of mindfulness that a study focuses on. When addressing specific outcomes that are suggested to be affected by mindfulness practice (e.g. sustained attention or rumination), control conditions should be adapted to this specific focus. The literature shows many examples of this guideline; most studies that investigated outcomes that were hypothesized to be affected by attentional focus have used control conditions in which participants were asked to think about whatever came to mind as opposed to focus on their breathing (e.g. Wilson et al., 2015). Clinically oriented studies addressing disengagement from negative thinking (decentering) have used control conditions in which participants are asked to focus on negative thoughts and to worry as opposed to focus on breathing (e.g. Arch & Craske, 2006). Alternatively, in emotion regulation research predominantly focusing on the acceptance component of mindfulness, control participants are typically asked to suppress rather than allow emotions to be present (e.g. Alberts et al., 2012).

Reducing demand and expectancy

As an inevitable consequence of the increased popularity of mindfulness, it is often hard if not impossible to prevent participants from knowing whether they are taking part in the mindfulness condition or the control condition. This can negatively affect the results of the study, for example, through experimenter demand, or through participants expecting and then experiencing or reporting certain benefits. Although it remains an unanswered question whether these problems can be fully circumvented, measures can be taken to at least reduce these unwanted effects. First, when recruiting participants for lab studies, advertisements and instructions should avoid the term "mindfulness" and instead use more general terms like "attention regulation". Second, longer-term mindfulness interventions should prevent or limit discussion of research findings, as this may raise expectations of participants. Preferably, the experimenter and trainer are not the same person, in order to prevent communication between participants and experimenter about the research.

Increasing adherence

Previous research has found that the total duration of formal home mindfulness practice, also referred to as mindfulness "dose effects", predicts positive outcomes like psychological symptom reduction, psychological well-being and perceived stress (Carmody & Baer, 2008). Although this relationship has not been reported by all studies (see for instance Carmody, Reed, Kristeller, & Merriam, 2008), it does suggest that it is important to maximize participants' adherence to instructions.

One way to increase adherence to instructions in lab settings is by facilitating mindfulness practice. Because many lab studies are conducted using students who often have no or little experience in mindfulness meditation, it is important to use clear, non-ambivalent instructions that have either been successfully used in previous research to induce mindfulness, or have been pretested. In addition, the circumstances under which participants are practicing mindfulness should be taken into consideration as well. By removing distractions (e.g. by turning off the lights) and increasing privacy (e.g. allowing participants to meditate without an experimenter watching them), adherence to the instructions in a lab session may be facilitated as well.

There are several possible ways to increase adherence in long-term interventions. First, during intake sessions, participants should be aware of the amount of training that is required during the intervention. Especially when daily practice is required, participants should confirm that they are willing and able to reserve time for home practice. In addition, when an intervention consists of plenary meetings, it must be clear how many sessions participants are required to attend.

Second, understanding of the requirements may be increased by offering participants booklets that clearly describe concrete homework assignments. Many participants have busy lives and often report that they simply "forgot" to practice. A possible way to overcome this problem is by sending daily reminders using mail or text messages. For instance, in a study by Alberts, Mulkens, Smeets, and Thewissen (2010), participants in the experimental group received a daily e-mail containing mindfulness quotes that were assumed to both increase commitment and remind participants of the intervention program. Third, practice may be enhanced by addressing the circumstances under which participants are practicing mindfulness at home. Informing family members about home practice can help to minimize interruptions during practice. Repeating a practice on regular bases using the same time and location is likely to result in a habit, which will lead to increased effects. Finally, for some people, starting with shorter mindfulness practice exercises and building from there is more effective in terms of adherence than starting with full 45-minute sessions.

Measuring compliance and adherence

As mentioned previously, often participants have little or no experience with mindfulness practice. In order to make sure that they comply with the instructions, brief manipulation check questionnaires have been used in lab studies. For instance, in a study by Campbell-Sills, Barlow, Brown, and Hofmann (2006), participants completed a 4-item, true/false questionnaire that tested their understanding of the instructions. In addition, a second manipulation check addressed how well participants were able to follow the audiotaped instructions. Another way to test whether a mindfulness manipulation was administered successfully is by using questionnaires that address state mindfulness. The state MAAS (Brown & Ryan, 2003) can be used to address whether a mindfulness induction has successfully resulted in an increased level of state mindfulness. Alternatively, the Toronto Mindfulness Scale (TMS, Lau et al., 2006) can be used to address mindfulness levels during practice.

In long-term interventions, registration of home practice time is typically used to measure adherence. Aside from gaining information about the level of engagement, this may also enhance commitment because participants are continually reminded of the importance of regular practice. Ideally, participants report practice time frequently, using experience sampling techniques that circumvent biased estimation of practice hours retrospectively. In a study by Goldin and Gross (2010), participants completed a self-report daily monitoring form each evening, recording both formal and informal meditation practices. Although daily measurements are preferred, asking participants for daily assessments on top of the weekly sessions and daily practice may introduce a practical challenge, especially when motivation is limited. In these cases, weekly measurements may be a suitable alternative for the more intensive daily assessments.

Discussion

As a result of the rapidly growing number of studies on mindfulness, the number of methods employed to investigate the concept have increased as well. The aim of the present chapter was to provide an overview of different methods to study mindfulness in the context of social psychology. Obviously, the current overview is far from complete. As an inevitable consequence of the large number of studies and the earlier addressed complexity of the construct, a selection was made of what are believed to be essential considerations when designing research on mindfulness.

As reflected by the great number of available self-report measures, an issue that warrants future attention is the creation of consensus regarding the exact meaning and underlying components of mindfulness. One possible route that may enhance our understanding about the multidimensional nature of mindfulness is the exploration of qualitative research. So far, only a few studies have used qualitative methods to study mindfulness. In an attempt to study the psychosocial aspects of mindfulness, Stanley and colleagues (2015) instructed participants to apply mindfulness (standing still, observing, etc.) in a busy, public place. Afterwards, participants were asked to describe what happened during the experiment, descriptively and in detail. Qualitative investigations may help to indicate the range of experiences that are likely to be encountered in a mindful state and at the same time reveal to which extent variation in findings arises through structural personal or social characteristics.

Another issue relates to the measurement of mindfulness. Mindfulness training has been found to decrease a narrative, descriptive and conceptually driven focus on the self and foster a more experiential focus, characterized by direct experience of sensation and emotion in the present moment (Farb et al., 2007). It remains an open question if this latter experience can be fully captured by methods that solely rely on descriptives and narratives, like questionnaires. In addition to self-report measures, the use of implicit measures may increase our understanding of processes that are influenced by mindfulness on an automatic and unconscious level (see for instance Barsalou, Chapter 3 in this volume). Linking these processes to explicit processes may reveal interesting resemblances or discrepancies between both. This may be especially relevant in a social context, where processes like stereotyping, self-esteem protection and social comparison have been found to operate at an unconscious level (see also Berry & Brown, Chapter 11 in this volume; Leary & Diebels, Chapter 4 in this volume).

To conclude, although there are still many gaps to be bridged in mindfulness research, the past years have offered a wide range of valuable tools and methods to approach the concept from a scientific angle. By critically assessing the literature and continuously exploring new ways to study and integrate the concept into existing fields of psychology, like social psychology, mindfulness is likely to continue establishing a stable position in the field of psychology.

References

Alberts, H. J. E. M., Mulkens, S., Smeets, M., & Thewissen, R. (2010). Coping with food cravings: Investigating the potential of a mindfulness-based intervention. *Appetite, 55,* 160–163.

Alberts, H. J. E. M., Schneider, F., & Martijn, C. (2012). Dealing efficiently with emotions: Acceptance-based coping with negative emotions requires fewer resources than suppression. *Cognition & Emotion, 26,* 863–870.

Alberts, H. J. E. M., & Thewissen, R. (2011). The effect of a brief mindfulness intervention on memory for positively and negatively valenced stimuli. *Mindfulness, 2,* 73–77.

Allen, M., Dietz, M., Blair, K. S., Van Beek, M., Rees, G., Vestergaard-Poulsen, P., . . . Roepstorff, A. (2012). Cognitive-affective neural plasticity following active-controlled mindfulness intervention. *Journal of Neuroscience, 32,* 15601–15610.

Arch, J. J., & Craske, M. G. (2006). Mechanisms of mindfulness: Emotion regulation following a focused breathing induction. *Behaviour Research and Therapy, 44,* 1849–1858.

Baer, R. A., Smith, G. T., & Allen, K. B. (2004). Assessment of mindfulness by self-report: The Kentucky inventory of mindfulness skills. *Assessment, 11*(3), 191–206.

Baer, R. A., Smith, G. T., Hopkins, J., Krietemeyer, J., & Toney, L. (2006). Using self-report assessment methods to explore facets of mindfulness. *Assessment, 13,* 27–45.

Bohlmeijer, E., ten Klooster, P. M., Fledderus, M., Veehof, M., & Baer, R. (2011). Psychometric properties of the five facet mindfulness questionnaire in depressed adults and development of a short form. *Assessment, 18,* 308–320.

Broderick, P. (2005). Mindfulness and coping with dysphoric mood: Contrasts with rumination and distraction. *Cognitive Therapy and Research, 29,* 501–510.

Brown, K. W., & Ryan, R. W. (2003). The benefits of being present: Mindfulness and its role in psychological well-being. *Journal of Personality and Social Psychology, 84,* 822–848.

Brown, K. W., Ryan, R. W., & Creswell, J. D. (2007). Mindfulness: Theoretical foundations and evidence for its salutary effects. *Psychological Inquiry, 18,* 211–237.

Call, D., Miron, L., & Orcutt, H. (2013). Effectiveness of brief mindfulness techniques in reducing symptoms of anxiety and stress. *Mindfulness, 5, 658–668.*

Campbell-Sills, L., Barlow, D. H., Brown, T. A., & Hofmann, S. G. (2006). Effects of suppression and acceptance on emotional responses of individuals with anxiety and mood disorders. *Behavior Research and Therapy, 40,* 1251–1262.

Cardaciotto, L. E., Herbert, J. D., Forman, M. E., Moitra, E., & Farrow, V. (2008). The assessment of present-moment awareness and acceptance. *Assessment, 15,* 204–223.

Carlson, L. E., Speca, M., Faris, P., & Patel, K. D. (2007). One year pre-post intervention follow-up of psychological, immune, endocrine and blood pressure outcomes of mindfulness-based stress reduction (MBSR) in breast and prostate cancer outpatients. *Brain Behavior and Immunity, 21,* 1038–1049.

Carmody, J., & Baer, R. A. (2008). Relationships between mindfulness practice and levels of mindfulness, medical and psychological symptoms and well-being in a mindfulness-based stress reduction program. *Journal of Behavioral Medicine, 31,* 23–33.

Carmody, J., Reed, G., Kristeller, J., & Merriam, P. (2008). Mindfulness, spirituality, and health-related symptoms. *Journal of Psychosomatic Research, 64,* 393–403.

Chambers, R., Chuen Yee Lo, B., & Allen, N. B. (2008). The impact of intensive mindfulness training on attentional control, cognitive style, and affect. *Cognitive Therapy and Research, 32,* 303–322.

Creswell, J. D., Way, B. M., Eisenberger, N. I., & Lieberman, M. D. (2007). Neural correlates of dispositional mindfulness during affect labeling. *Psychosomatic Medicine, 69,* 560–565.

Dekeyser, M., Raes, F., Leijssen, M., Leysen, S., & Dewulf, D. (2008). Mindfulness skills and interpersonal behaviour. *Personality and Individual Differences, 44,* 1235–1245.

Duval, S., & Wicklund, R. A. (1972). *A theory of objective self-awareness.* New York: Academic Press.

Erisman, S. M., & Roemer, L. (2010). A preliminary investigation of the effects of experimentally induced mindfulness on emotional responding to film clips. *Emotion, 10,* 72–82.

Farb, N. A. S., Segal, Z. V., Mayberg, H., Bean, J., McKeon, D., Fatima, Z., & Anderson, A. K. (2007). Attending to the present: Mindfulness meditation reveals distinct neural modes of self-reference. *Social Cognitive and Affective Neuroscience, 2,* 313–122.

Feldman, G., Hayes, A., Kumar, S., Greeson, J., & Laurenceau, J. P. (2007). Mindfulness and emotion regulation: The development and initial validation of the Cognitive and Affective Mindfulness Scale-Revised (CAMS-R). *Journal of Psychopathology and Behavioral Assessment, 29,* 177–190.

Flook, L., Goldberg, S. B., Pinger, L., & Davidson, R. J. (2015). Promoting prosocial behavior and self-regulatory skills in preschool children through a mindfulness-based kindness curriculum. *Developmental Psychology, 51,* 44–51.

Frewen, P. A., Evans, E., Maraj, N., Dozois, D. J. A., & Partridge, K. (2008). Letting go: Mindfulness and negative automatic thinking. *Cognitive Therapy & Research, 32,* 758–774.

Garland, E. L., Hanley, A., Farb, N. A., & Froeliger, B. (2013). State mindfulness during meditation predicts enhanced cognitive reappraisal. *Mindfulness, 6,* 234–243.

Germer, C. K. (2005). Anxiety disorders: Befriending fear. In C. K. Germer, R. D. Siegel, & P. R. Fulton (Eds.), *Mindfulness and psychotherapy* (pp. 152–172). New York: Guilford Press.

Goldin, P. R., & Gross, J. J. (2010). Effects of mindfulness-based stress reduction (MBSR) on emotion regulation in social anxiety disorder. *Emotion, 10,* 83–91.

Greco, L. A., Baer, R. A., & Smith, G. T. (2011). Supplemental material for assessing mindfulness in children and adolescents: Development and validation of the Child and Adolescent Mindfulness Measure (CAMM). *Psychological Assessment, 23,* 606–614.

Grossman, P. (2008). On measuring mindfulness in psychosomatic and psychological research. *Journal of Psychosomatic Research, 64,* 405–408.

Hölzel, B. K., Ott, U., Gard, T., Hempel, H., Weygandt, M., Morgen, K., & Vaitl, D. (2008). Investigation of mindfulness meditation practitioners with voxel-based morphometry. *Social Cognitive and Affective Neuroscience, 3,* 55–61.

Hulsheger, U., Alberts, H. J. E. M., Feinhold, A., & Lang, J. W. B. (2012). Benefits of mindfulness at work: The role of mindfulness in emotion regulation, emotional exhaustion, and job satisfaction. *Journal of Applied Psychology, 98,* 310–325.

Jennings, S. J., & Jennings, J. L. (2013). Peer-directed, brief mindfulness training with adolescents: A pilot study. *International Journal of Behavioral Consultation and Therapy, 8,* 23–25.

Kabat-Zinn, J. (1982). An out-patient program in behavioral medicine for chronic pain patients based on the practice of mindfulness meditation: Theoretical considerations and preliminary results. *General Hospital Psychiatry, 4,* 33–47.

Kabat-Zinn, J. (1990). *Full catastrophe living: Using the wisdom of your body and mind to face stress, pain and illness*. New York: Delacorte.

Keefe, T. (1979). The development of empathic skills: A study. *Journal of Education for Social Work, 15*, 10–14.

Kuehner, C., Huffziger, S., & Liebsch, K. (2009). Rumination, distraction and mindful self-focus: Effects on mood, dysfunctional attitudes and cortisol stress response. *Psychological Medicine, 39*, 219–228.

Lau, M. A., Bishop, S. R., Segal, Z. V., Buis, T., Anderson, N. D., Carlson, L., . . . Devins, G. (2006). The Toronto mindfulness scale: Development and validation. *Journal of Clinical Psychology, 62*, 1445–1467.

Lueke, A., & Gibson, B. (2014). Mindfulness meditation reduces implicit age and race bias: The role of reduced automaticity of responding. *Social Psychological and Personality Science, 6*, 284–291.

Michalak, J., Heidenreich, T., Meibert, P., & Schulte, D. (2008). Mindfulness predicts relapse/recurrence in major depressive disorder following mindfulness-based cognitive therapy. *Journal of Nervous and Mental Disease, 196*, 630–633.

Mrazek, M. D., Franklin, M. S., Phillips, D., Baird, B., & Schooler, J. (2013). Mindfulness training improves working memory and GRE performance while reducing mind-wandering. *Psychological Science, 24*, 776–781.

Mrazek, M. D., Smallwood, J., & Schooler, J. W. (2012). Mindfulness and mind-wandering: finding convergence through opposing constructs. *Emotion, 12*(3), 442–448.

Oman, D., Shapiro, S. L., Thoresen, C. E., Plante, T. G., & Flinders, T. (2008). Meditation lowers stress and supports forgiveness among college students: A randomized controlled trial. *Journal of American College Health, 56*, 569–578.

Ortner, C. M. N., Kilner, S., & Zelazo, P. D. (2007). Mindfulness meditation and emotional interference in a simple cognitive task. *Motivation and Emotion, 31*, 271–283.

Pepping, C. A., O'Donovan, A., Zimmer-Gembeck, M. J., & Hanisch, M. (2014). Is emotion regulation the process underlying the relationship between low mindfulness and psychosocial distress? *Australian Journal of Psychology, 66*(2), 130–138.

Ramsey, L. T., & Jones, E. E. (2015). Minding the interpersonal gap: Mindfulness-based interventions in the prevention of ostracism. *Consciousness and Cognition, 31*, 24–34.

Schmertz, S. K., Anderson, P. L., & Robins, D. L. (2009). The relation between self-report mindfulness and performance on tasks of sustained attention. *Journal of Psychopathology and Behavioral Assessment, 31*, 60–66.

Segal, Z. V., Williams, J. M. G., & Teasdale, J. D. (2002). *Mindfulness-based cognitive therapy for depression*. New York: Guilford Press.

Shaver, P. R., Lavy, S., Saron, C. D., & Mikulincer, M. (2007). Social foundations of the capacity for mindfulness: An attachment perspective. *Psychological Inquiry: An international Journal for the Advancement of Psychological Theory, 18*, 264–271.

Stanley, S., Barker, M., Edwards, V., & McEwen, E. (2015). Swimming against the Stream? Mindfulness as a psychosocial research methodology. *Qualitative Research in Psychology, 12*, 61–76.

Tan, L. B. G., Lo, B. C. Y., & Macrae, C. N. (2014). Brief mindfulness meditation improves mental state attribution and empathizing. *PLoS ONE, 9*, e110510. doi:10.1371/journal.pone.0110510

Tang, Y-Y., Hölzel, B. K., & Posner, M. I. (2015). The neuroscience of mindfulness meditation. *Nature Reviews Neuroscience, 16*, 213–225.

Taylor, V. A., Grant, J., Daneault, V., Scavone, G., Breton, E., Roffe-Vidal, S., . . . Beauregard, M. (2011). Impact of mindfulness on the neural responses to emotional pictures in experienced and beginner meditators. *Neuroimage, 57*, 1524–1533.

Van Doesum, N. J., Van Lange, D. A. W., & Van Lange, P. A. M. (2013). Social mindfulness: Skill and will to navigate the social world. *Journal of Personality and Social Psychology, 105,* 86–103.

Vinchurkar, S. A., Singh, D., & Visweswaraiah, N. K. (2014). Self-reported measures of mindfulness in meditators and non-meditators: A cross-sectional study. *International Journal of Yoga, 7,* 142–146.

Wilson, B. M., Mickes, L., Stolarz-Fantino, S., Evrard, M., & Fantino, E. (2015). Increased false-memory susceptibility after mindfulness meditation. *Psychological Science, 26,* 1567–1573.

3

UNDERSTANDING CONTEMPLATIVE PRACTICES FROM THE PERSPECTIVE OF DUAL-PROCESS THEORIES

Lawrence W. Barsalou

Dual-process theories

From the dual-process perspective, psychological phenomena typically include: (1) impulsive and habitual processes that are relatively involuntary, implicit, and unconscious, often associated with hedonic short-term goals, requiring few executive resources; and (2) regulatory and reflective processes that are relatively voluntary, explicit, and conscious, often associated with rational long-term goals, requiring significant use of executive resources. For any given psychological phenomenon, the basic idea is that initial processing results from the first type of process, with the second type of process available optionally to regulate it.

Dual-process theories have played central roles in explaining cognitive, social, affective, and appetitive phenomena for decades. At least since James (1890/1950), cognitive psychologists have incorporated the dual-process framework extensively into their theory and research (e.g. Evans, 1984; Posner & Snyder, 1975; Schneider & Shiffrin, 1977; Sloman, 1996). Social psychologists have similarly incorporated the dual-process framework extensively into their work (e.g. Chaiken & Trope, 1999; Metcalfe & Mischel, 1999; Sherman, Gawronski, & Trope, 2014; Strack & Deutsch, 2004). In a major review of dual-process theories, Stanovich and West (2000) dubbed the two processes of dual-process theories "System 1" and "System 2." Given the ubiquity of these two kinds of processes across human behaviour, they are likely to be important in contemplative practices as well.

A fundamental assumption of many dual-process theories is that System 1 causes the lion's share of behaviour, emotion, and thought. From this perspective, daily experience in the world conditions the associative structures in memory that produce actions, bodily states, and cognitive processing. Furthermore, System 2 has relatively little control over behaviour, emotion, and thought (e.g. Goschke, 2013), while creating intuitive theories about oneself and the world via language, social interaction, and culture that are often limited and incorrect (e.g. Wilson, 2004).

Significant implications for measurement follow from dual-process assumptions about behavioural causes and intuitive theories (e.g. Gawronski & Payne, 2011; Greenwald & Banaji, 1995). In psychological research, it has become widely accepted that explicit self-report measures are unlikely to measure the causal mechanisms of interest in System 1 accurately. Because people typically have little conscious access to the System 1 mechanisms that cause their behaviour, emotion, and thought, they have little ability to know and describe these mechanisms accurately. Instead, self-report measures are much more likely to capture people's intuitive theories about these causes in System 2. To accurately measure the mechanisms in System 1 requires the use of implicit measures that target System 1 mechanisms indirectly without people's awareness.

Thus, from the dual-process perspective, System 1 constitutes a huge system of conditioned mechanisms that operate largely unconsciously, often producing behaviour, emotion, and thought outside deliberate control, in relatively automatic and habitual manners. Because it often feels as if an out-of-control beast occupies our brain and runs our life, System 1 is sometimes referred to metaphorically as a *10,000-pound gorilla*. Nevertheless, System 2 offers significant resources for regulating System 1's activity. Once System 1 begins to produce an action, for example, System 2 can inhibit it or replace it with another action. In humans, the executive system underlies the ability to self-regulate, capitalizing on significantly expanded frontal and associative systems in the brain (e.g. Berger, 2011; Buckner & Krienen, 2013; Goschke, 2013; Hofmann, Schmeichel, & Baddeley, 2012; Mischel et al., 2011). Besides regulating behaviour, emotion, and thought in the current moment, regulatory processes can attempt to implement long-term changes well into the future (e.g. Stanovich, West, & Toplak, 2014; Wilson, 2011).

Challenges to dual-process theories

Much theory and research make it clear that reifying Systems 1 and 2 into two distinct systems is unjustified (e.g. Moors & De Houwer, 2006; Sharma, Markon, & Clark, 2014; Stahl et al., 2014; also see relevant chapters in Sherman et al., 2014). One problem is that processes associated with System 1 are highly diverse, as are processes associated with System 2, suggesting that neither kind of process originates in a fixed system. Conversely, processes associated with System 1 often share properties with processes associated with System 2, further suggesting that the two kinds of processes don't originate in different rigid systems.

A much more plausible approach is to simply assume that brain architecture in humans has evolved to produce what I will call *Involuntary Initial Responses* (IRs) and *Optional Regulatory Responses* (RRs).[1] IRs reflect the basic neural architecture of ascending pathways in modality-specific systems. As a stimulus is perceived (e.g. in vision, audition, taste), its sensory and perceptual features are processed early in these pathways, followed by conceptual processing later. During conceptual processing, multimodal patterns may be accessed that produce inferences about the stimulus, including its value for the perceiver and actions that the perceiver could perform on it. Because most stimuli have become conditioned in this manner, perceiving just about anything in the environment is likely to produce some kind of IR.[2]

Conversely, RRs reflect the ability to regulate IRs using diverse meta-cognitive and regulatory abilities. Because the human brain has been endowed with large association areas and frontal lobes, humans can regulate their responses to stimuli in a flexible manner. Although IRs occur constantly, humans have the ability to monitor these responses, evaluate them, and then inhibit, change, or protect them.

Implications of dual-process theories for contemplative practices

The dual-process perspective fits naturally with contemplative approaches. Given how broadly the dual-process perspective applies to cognitive and social phenomena, it's not surprising that it applies to contemplative approaches, too. Here, I focus on Buddhism, because mindfulness – the focus of this edited volume – plays such a central role in it. I also focus on Buddhism because it's the only contemplative approach that I know anything about (in particular, Tibetan Buddhism). Because I'm *far* from an expert, however, my discussions of Buddhism should be viewed as simply attempting to offer a general and relatively superficial account of how the dual-process perspective can be brought to bear on contemplative practices.

First, consider The Four Noble Truths that lie at the core of Buddhism (e.g. Gethin, 2010), described here from the Western perspective. According to the First Noble Truth, life contains considerable suffering, which not only includes physical suffering such as hardship, disease, and loss, but also extensive psychological suffering, related to grasping and aversion (e.g. stress, negative emotion, dissatisfaction). According to the Second Noble Truth, one important source of psychological suffering is the conditioning of a person's cognitive system, which produces constant grasping and aversion. For example, frequently craving sweets, eating too many, and then feeling guilty about consuming them results from years of conditioning that produce appetitive desires for sweets in general, inability to regulate their consumption, and dysfunctional emotional sequelae. According to the Third Noble Truth, reducing the psychological suffering that one experiences is possible. By changing the conditioning that causes suffering, a happier and healthier life can result. According to the Fourth Noble Truth, various practices and strategies exist for changing one's conditioning, which take advantage of the inherent flexibility and potential for change in human nature. Intentionally becoming mindful of impulses to consume sweets, for example, and learning to watch these impulses dissipate without acting on them can lead to improvements in physical and psychological well-being (see Papies, Chapter 7 in this volume).

From the dual-process perspective, the First and Second Noble Truths bear on the conditioning responsible for behaviour, emotion, and thought, whereas the Third and Fourth Noble Truths bear on the potential for acquiring strategies that regulate and change this conditioning. As we will see later, the Fourth Noble Truth is associated with the Eight-Fold Path, which is a sophisticated collection of regulatory strategies capable of transforming every aspect of a person's life, including their cognition, affect, ethics, actions, self, and subjective experience.

The fundamental principle of karma in Buddhism offers a related example. According to this principle, a person's intentions and actions condition their character, habits, and subjective experience (e.g. Gethin, 2010). Because karma reflects all the conditioning that a person has accumulated over a lifetime (and over previous lifetimes if one accepts reincarnation), it is the 10,000-pound gorilla that dominates behaviour, emotion, and thought via IRs. The construct of karma fits quite comfortably with the dual-process assumption that conditioning governs people's existence. Within this conditioning, a wide variety of RRs may also be available, such as adopting contemplative (and other regulatory) practices that change one's conditioning for the better.

IRs in contemplative practices

As we just saw, the Four Noble Truths state that a person's conditioning is responsible for their suffering. Buddhism offers many further proposals on the nature of suffering, describing in some detail the conditioning that makes people unhappy. In general, people suffer because they live in samsara, the psychological world of illusion and dissatisfaction. As they experience entities and events in their daily activities, they react to them cognitively and emotionally in ways that throw them off balance, such that they do not experience happiness (e.g. Ricard, 2007).

From the dual-process perspective, these non-optimal reactions can be viewed as the consequences of IRs. As entities and events are encountered in the world, they activate IRs via past conditioning that produce imbalance and unhappiness, often in relatively subtle ways. Although IRs serve a wide variety of useful goals in daily life, they may not necessarily lead to balance and happiness. On seeing a tasty food, for example, the IRs that cause people to approach and consume it ensure that they won't starve. The downside, though, is that these IRs also cause desire and craving, which make people dissatisfied, wanting things they don't currently have. Furthermore, these desires and craving, if acted on inappropriately, can eventually lead to outcomes that make people unhappy and unhealthy, such as becoming overweight or diabetic.

According to Buddhism, several important types of IR underlie dissatisfaction and unhappiness: grasping and aversion, the illusion of self, negative emotions, and mind-wandering. The following subsections address each in turn. A final subsection further notes that RRs have the potential to exacerbate the problems that IRs initiate (before turning to the final section to how RRs can instead ameliorate these problems).

Grasping and aversion

Many traditions of Buddhism assume that several *root causes* underlie people's dissatisfaction and unhappiness, permeating the conditioning that controls their behaviour (e.g. Bodhi, 2005; Gethin, 2010). Two of these root causes are grasping and aversion. Whereas grasping is the desire to possess something, aversion is the desire to avoid something. In each case, a desire emerges for something other than the current state of affairs. Most importantly, the current moment is viewed as lacking in some way, creating an imbalance that leads to dissatisfaction and unhappiness (e.g. Gethin, 2010; Loy, 2002). The extensive suffering and samsara that people experience, as noted in the Four Noble Truths, results from this lack and imbalance that they experience constantly in their lives. As people continually grasp at some things and attempt to avoid others, they create a perpetual sense of unease and are never truly happy.

From the dual-process perspective, the constant grasping and aversion that people experience can be viewed as resulting from the constant activation of IRs. As entities and events are encountered in the world (or imagined in thought), they trigger IRs that produce tendencies to approach them (grasping) or to avoid them (aversion). In the terms of Western science, grasping leads to approach behaviour associated with positive valence, whereas aversion leads to avoidance behaviour associated with negative valence. In this way, the Buddhist constructs of grasping and aversion map naturally onto the central scientific constructs of approach and avoidance, and also onto those for positive and negative valence (cf. Barrett & Bliss-Moreau, 2009).

Extensive scientific research demonstrates that entities and events generally activate a wide variety of valenced responses. The evaluative priming task in social psychology, for example, demonstrates that words and pictures often produce evaluative responses as IRs, some positive and some negative (for a review, see Herring et al., 2013). Typically, evaluative priming research focuses on words and pictures that produce strong evaluative responses (e.g. baby, robbery). Arguably, however, there is no such thing as a completely neutral response to anything (e.g. sparrow, television; Lebrecht, Bar, Barrett, & Tarr, 2012). In general, these widespread evaluative responses can be viewed as tendencies to approach and avoid the respective stimuli, or in Buddhist terms, as tendencies for grasping and aversion.

Increasing neuroscience research similarly demonstrates that perceiving stimuli activates brain areas quickly that produce evaluations, especially the orbital-frontal cortex (OFC). When viewing visual objects briefly, for example, not only does visual processing of the object occur, so does rapid evaluative processing (e.g. Chaumon, Kveraga, Barrett, & Bar, 2014; Lebrecht et al., 2012; Shenhav, Barrett, & Bar, 2012). Within much less than a second of viewing an object, the brain produces an evaluation of it, often unconsciously (e.g. Hermans, De Houwer, & Eelen, 2001; Winkielman, Berridge, & Wilbarger, 2005). As extensive literature shows, evaluative responses are produced to just about everything, with different domains of evaluative responses residing in domain-specific areas of OFC (Rudebeck & Murray, 2014; Wilson, Takahashi, Schoenbaum, & Niv, 2014).

Thus, the Buddhist proposal that grasping and avoidance lie at the heart of human conditioning finds strong support from both behavioural and neuroscience research. One of the most basic things that people do is to evaluate whether the entities and events they encounter are good or bad, and whether they should approach or avoid them.

Finally, the strong impulses and desires that people often experience can be highly disruptive to mental, physical, and social well-being. Because these particular IRs are especially intense and compelling, they may often have the most potent motivational effects on ensuing behaviour (e.g. Papies & Barsalou, 2015; Papies, Pronk, Keesman, & Barsalou, 2015). For this reason, developing good regulatory strategies, such as mindfulness, may be especially important for managing impulses and desires. To the extent that intense IRs can arise and dissipate without affecting behaviour, they become less likely to produce problems, such that greater control and choice emerge.

The illusion of self

As described in the previous section, Buddhism assumes that several root causes lie at the heart of people's conditioning, with two of these being grasping and aversion. The most important root cause, however, is *the illusion of self* (e.g. Bodhi, 2005; Gethin, 2010). As Buddhists often note, people experience a self inside them. Not only does this *self* seem to be who they are, it is also the self who makes things happen, to whom things happen, who evaluates things, and so forth. As Buddhists further note, this self is really just a cognitive construction that doesn't exist anywhere other than in people's minds. Western scientists who study the self often agree (e.g. Baumeister, 1998; Northoff et al., 2006; see Leary and Diebels, Chapter 4 in this volume).

According to Buddhism, this illusory sense of self constitutes the most central aspect of human conditioning, lying at the heart of people's dissatisfaction and unhappiness. It is the most basic root of samsara, ultimately responsible for the constant grasping and aversion that people exhibit over the course of daily activity. Because people are so invested in promoting and protecting their sense of self, they constantly grasp at things that they believe will promote it, and constantly avoid things they believe will harm it. Every entity and event encountered becomes evaluated with respect to one's self-interests, with grasping and aversion being the outcomes of these evaluations.

The constant sense of self that people experience can be viewed as resulting from IRs. Based on a lifetime of conditioning, people develop a huge amount of knowledge about who they believe they are, with aspects of this knowledge becoming active dynamically in a context-dependent manner when relevant (e.g. Markus & Wurf, 1987). As people encounter entities and events, the conditioned IRs that result can include senses of self, thereby carrying information about one's self-interests in an implicit manner. Not only do IRs represent an evaluation of an entity or event, but they also represent how it bears on one's self-interests. These senses of self can reflect diverse sources of self-related information, including one's goals, values, and traits, together with the in-groups to which one belongs and their associated norms (e.g. Baumeister, 1998; Frable, 1997; Markus & Wurf, 1987).

Much evidence in neuroscience demonstrates that a large distributed network along the cortical midline, from ventral and dorsal prefrontal areas to the posterior cingulate, becomes active to process self-relevance (e.g. Northoff et al., 2006). As people view a wide variety of self-relevant stimuli (e.g. traits, faces, scenes), this network becomes active to process them. Interestingly, these same areas become active to process other individuals besides oneself, suggesting that processing the self-related interests of others is not only important, but also draws on the same general system that processes information about oneself. Sui, Humphreys, and their colleagues have recently provided a large body of especially compelling evidence for the significant power of self-relevance (e.g. Sui & Humphreys, 2015a, 2015b; Sui, Liu, Mevorach, & Humphreys, 2015; Sui, Rotshtein, & Humphreys, 2013). Simply associating a random shape with oneself, for example, makes the shape much more salient and relevant than usual. Not only does the shape become more important conceptually, it becomes easier to process perceptually. In summary, all of these neural and behavioural findings make it clear that self-related processing constitutes a central part of cognition, as Buddhist assumptions about the root causes of conditioning anticipate.

Notably, however, Western science doesn't view self-related processing with the same antipathy as does Buddhism. To the contrary, self-related processing is often viewed much more positively in Western traditions, such that Western science is less oriented to examining how self-related processing produces dissatisfaction and unhappiness. Thus, an important issue for future research is reconciling this tension regarding the positive versus negative effects of self.

Destructive emotions

As we have seen, bottom-up processing continually produces IRs to entities and events encountered during daily activity. Not surprisingly, the initial evaluations and self-assessments in these IRs can lead to increasingly complex, powerful, and temporally extended emotions. As the implications of an important entity or event become clear, a strong emotional response is likely to signal this importance and to motivate relevant actions for some time thereafter. Rather than simply experiencing the entity or event with equanimity and letting it pass, people often experience it with extended emotion that reflects self-interested grasping and/or aversion, perpetuated through rumination. Not only does such emotion throw people out of balance, it may also lead to actions that are dysfunctional or destructive. When a friend disapproves of your clothing, for example, the self-interested aversion that results may produce anger, followed by a desire for revenge that leads to reciprocal disapproval.

The construct of destructive emotion plays a central role in Buddhism, being contrasted with constructive emotion (e.g. Dreyfus, 2008; Goleman, 2003). Destructive emotion is the natural consequence of self-interest, grasping, and aversion; it plays salient and central roles in the dissatisfaction and unhappiness that constitutes samsara; and it can lead to destructive intentions and actions. In Western science, the closely related constructed of *neuroticism* is typically associated with experiencing extensive amounts of negative emotion. As much research shows, increasing neuroticism is strongly associated with increased health problems, increased social problems, decreased psychological well-being, and lower longevity (e.g. Lahey, 2009).

Again, both Buddhism and Western science converge. To the extent that destructive/negative emotion results from IRs to entities and events in the world, quality of life decreases. Again, however, important differences exist. Westerners, for example, view pride as a positive emotion that reflects a strong self, whereas Buddhists view it as a negative emotion that destroys equanimity (i.e. by grasping at the things that motivate feeling proud).

Mind-wandering

As IRs produce evaluations, self-related responses, and emotions, they can further launch thought into mental time travel, taking people out of the current moment as they imagine being in some other situation. Rather than focusing on the task at hand, people become preoccupied with their thoughts. Seeing a friend, for example, might produce an IR related to their recent disapproval, which causes re-enactment of the previous situation, followed by planning further revenge in the near future. In the process, awareness of the present situation fades, as has any equanimity that might have existed. Instead, grasping and aversion at past and future events take over, motivated by self-interest.

The dysfunctional roles of mind-wandering have been noted widely both in contemplative traditions (e.g. Dreyfus, 2011; Dunne, 2011; Fronsdal, 2001; Kabat-Zinn, 1994) and in Western science (e.g. Hofmann, Baumeister, Förster, & Vohs, 2012; Kane & McVay, 2012; Killingsworth & Gilbert, 2010; Lutz, Jha, Dunne, & Saron, 2015; Mrazek et al., 2012). Certainly mind-wandering can be productive when people are planning future events, solving problems, and so forth (e.g. Baird, Smallwood, & Schooler, 2011; Gerlach, Spreng, Madore, & Schacter, 2014). Nevertheless, mind-wandering can also produce distractions that lead to performance errors in external tasks, psychopathology through rumination, and so forth. Regardless, mind-wandering, at least to some extent, can again be viewed as the sequelae of IRs.

Finally, the brain areas that produce mind-wandering in the default mode network overlap extensively with the brain areas that process self-relevance (e.g. Kucyi & Davis, 2014; Mittner et al., 2014; Qin & Northoff, 2011; Sheline et al., 2009). Such findings strongly suggest that mind-wandering often focuses on self-related interests, consistent with self-absorption being the root cause of dissatisfaction and unhappiness in Buddhism.

Exacerbating IRs with RRs

At some point as an IR evolves from evaluation to mind-wandering, regulatory processing may take over. As we will see in the next section, regulatory processing could attempt to down regulate an IR via inhibition, reappraisal, mindfulness, and so forth. On some occasions, however, regulatory processing might instead exacerbate the problems that an IR initiates by up-regulating the evaluation, self-related processing, and emotion that occurs. When encountering an appetitive stimulus, such as a food or a drug, an initial IR might produce an approach tendency toward it. Rather than down-regulating the IR, however, a subsequent RR could up-regulate it into a full-blown craving, creating a temporally extended obsession to consume the appetitive object (e.g. Kavanagh, Andrade, & May, 2005). In this manner, RRs have the potential to significantly increase the evaluations, self-relevance, and emotion associated with processing an entity or event, thereby increasing the problems that regulatory processing in contemplative practices aims to address.

RRs in contemplative practices

Contemplative practices, such as Buddhism, typically recognize that they have a 10,000-pound gorilla on their hands, and then set out to do something about it. As we have seen, Buddhism first analyzes the problem, focusing on the nature of the underlying causal system that produces the problematic behaviour, emotion, and thought. By understanding the problem, it becomes possible to formulate a solution that effectively targets the critical mechanisms. In Buddhism, the solution can be viewed as an attempt to implement RRs that, first, manage problematic IRs and their root causes, and second, replace them with a causal system that produces healthier IRs.

Consistent with dual-process theories, Buddhism implements short-term RRs that manage problematic IRs in the moment, together with long-term RRs that produce significant long-term change in behaviour, emotion, and thought (e.g. Stanovich et al., 2014). Together, these RRs attempt to tame self-interest, grasping, aversion, destructive emotion, and mind-wandering, and to replace them with a positive set of qualities, such as selflessness, kindness, generosity, and compassion. Should a practitioner be successful, their experience of life shifts increasingly from samsara to equanimity and happiness.

In the next subsections, after discussing how RRs are learned and implemented (assembling RRs), we will consider various RRs in Buddhism that attempt to: (1) manage problematic IRs in the moment (concentration and mindfulness practices), (2) replace problematic IRs with new IRs over the long-term (conduct practices), (3) fundamentally restructure a person's subjective experience of mind (wisdom practices). Together, these three kinds of contemplative practices constitute the Eight-Fold Path in Buddhism, an impressive collection of regulatory strategies that aim to transform a person's mindfulness, ethical conduct, and wisdom, respectively (e.g. Gethin, 2010). From the dual-process perspective, these contemplative practices establish a wide variety of RRs, some that manage IRs in the moment, and others that attempt long-term change. For a review of these three types of contemplative practice from the perspective of Western science and clinical practice, see Dahl, Lutz, and Davidson (2015). Here, the focus is on how the dual-process approach produces insight into these practices.

Assembling RRs

Initially, when a new contemplative practice is acquired (e.g. mindfulness, compassion), RRs are required to learn and implement it. Because the practice hasn't been encoded into IRs, it can't yet run implicitly in the background, but instead requires deliberate control. With regular practice, however, IRs develop to implement the practice more implicitly, such that it increasingly runs in the background, without the use of regulatory resources.

Importantly, however, people don't learn contemplative practices completely from scratch. Instead, their cognitive systems already possess many of the basic abilities relevant to performing these strategies, such that initially learning a contemplative practice primarily involves assembling existing abilities into new RRs (e.g. Bishop et al., 2006; Lebois et al., 2015). One source of evidence for this hypothesis is the finding that non-meditators can be taught simple beginning contemplative skills in as little as 10–15 minutes. Specifically, participants can quickly begin to acquire concentration skills associated with mindfulness (e.g. Dickenson, Berkman, Arch, & Lieberman, 2013), as well as decentering skills (e.g. Lebois et al., 2015; Papies, Barsalou, & Custers, 2012; Papies et al., 2015; Tincher, Lebois, & Barsalou, 2015). Initial – albeit superficial – learning of these skills can occur quickly because they draw on existing cognitive processes such as strategic attention and perspective shifting. Thus, learning a contemplative practice is not a mysterious esoteric practice, but a natural and relatively transparent assembly of existing abilities, at least initially.

No doubt, extensive practice that transforms RRs into IRs is essential for realizing the full potential of contemplative practices, or to even begin experiencing a significant fraction of their potential. Furthermore, extensive practice is likely to create new cognitive skills that didn't exist previously. Nevertheless, early practice appears to build upon and benefit significantly from pre-existing processing resources that can be assembled into new RRs.

Concentration and mindfulness practices

A basic (often preliminary) contemplative practice on the Eight-Fold Path simply involves improving the abilities to concentrate and be mindful. One common technique is to practice holding attention on something continually, such as on the breath or an external object (e.g. Kornbloom, 2008; Salzberg, 2011). Over time, properly performed practice increases the duration of how long concentration can be maintained. Because concentrating on a variety of instructions, texts, mental states, and so forth is essential for properly performing later contemplative practices on the Eight-Fold Path, developing the ability to concentrate is an important first step. For an account of the neural networks assembled to perform this practice, see Hasenkamp, Wilson-Mendenhall, Duncan, and Barsalou (2012).

As concentration strengthens, mindfulness typically increases (e.g. Kabat-Zinn, 1994; Kornbloom, 2008; Salzberg, 2011). While attempting to concentrate on an object, attention invariably drifts away, as the practitioner's mind wanders. Learning to understand and handle mind-wandering is arguably the crux of concentration and mindfulness practices. The first step in developing mindfulness is to realize that attention has wandered away from the focal object. The second step is to recognize the nature of the distraction without evaluating it or reacting in some way (remaining non-evaluative and non-reactive; Kabat-Zinn, 1994). The third step is returning attention to the object of concentration. For related but different forms of mindfulness practice, see Dreyfus (2011) and Dunne (2011, 2015).

Together, the RRs assembled to implement concentration and mindfulness practices begin to disable problematic IRs. By developing RRs that increase concentration, it becomes possible to simply observe IRs as they arise, such that they are less likely to control cognition, emotion, and action unconsciously. As a result, the practitioner begins to better see the grasping, aversion, self-processing, and emotion that IRs produce. By developing RRs that enforce non-evaluation and non-reactivity, the practitioner learns to experience IRs without evaluating and acting on them. Rather than producing extended emotion and action, IRs simply arise and dissipate. In this manner, mindfulness begins to break the karmic cycle. Not engaging with an IR stops the normal process of perpetuating it as a habit and entrenching it further as a causal mechanism in a bottom-up pathway. Instead, the IR becomes increasingly ineffective every time it is experienced mindfully, thereby decreasing its future likelihood of becoming active and affecting behaviour, emotion, and thought.

With increasing practice, mindfulness has the potential to alter a wide variety of IRs associated with grasping, aversion, and self-relevance. To the extent that these IRs no longer govern mental experience, dissatisfaction with the current state of the world becomes less likely. Once the world no longer appears lacking in some way, increasingly extended states of equanimity follow, leading to happiness (e.g. Ricard, 2007).

A frequent misunderstanding about mindfulness is that the equanimity it produces causes people to withdraw from the world. To the contrary, mindfulness leads to freedom from the problematic IRs that normally control cognition, emotion, and action. When problematic IRs no longer dominate consciousness, greater choice in how to act becomes possible. Indeed, some mindfulness practices stress the importance of engaging in ethical evaluation of mind-wandering states for the purpose of evaluating the character of one's intentions and potential actions (e.g. Dreyfus, 2011; Dunne, 2011, 2015). From this perspective, it is necessary to evaluate the ethical implications of one's distracting thoughts for the purpose of personal growth. Thus, mindfulness isn't simply a tool for achieving the peace of equanimity – although that is certainly a benefit – it can also play central roles in making the practitioner a better person and a positive force in the world through wiser decisions and actions (see Condon, Chapter 9 in this volume). Indeed, many Western mindfulness practitioners become increasingly engaged in addressing social problems (e.g. socially engaged Buddhism; see King, 2009).

Finally, the dual-process perspective offers a potentially useful framework for understanding the regulatory processes that underlie concentration and mindfulness practices. The large theoretical and empirical literatures associated with self-regulation offer explanatory systems for understanding how these practices are learned initially and begin to produce positive effects. Specifically, these practices can be viewed as drawing heavily on classic attention mechanisms for focusing, shifting, disengagement, and vigilance (cf. Chun, Golomb, & Turk-Browne, 2011; Thompson, Besner, & Smilek, 2015). In addition, these practices draw heavily on the executive system and its ability to regulate cognition, emotion, and action through goal setting, plan execution, goal protection, inhibition, and so forth (e.g. Berger, 2011; Goschke, 2013; Hofmann et al., 2012; Mischel et al., 2011).

Conduct practices

As we just saw, developing concentration and mindfulness creates space for new attitudes, intentions, and behaviours to develop. The second major set of practices on the Eight-Fold-Path – conduct practices – take advantage of this space, aiming to restructure the bottom-up pathways that initially control behaviour, emotion, and thought through IRs. As this restructuring occurs, it increasingly changes how the practitioner experiences the world and acts in it. As a consequence of performing conduct practices, the practitioner becomes less selfish, more oriented towards others, and more ethical. Not only do these changes in perspective increase a person's social contributions, but they also make them happier (e.g. Dunne, 2015; Ricard, 2007). Happiness cannot occur without these changes: Equanimity is not enough.

Lojong in Tibetan Buddhism constitutes one classic form of conduct practice, often referred to as *mind training* (e.g. Jinpa, 2006). The core material of Lojong is transmitted through a variety of texts that include slogans, aphorisms, and verses. As practitioners study and learn from these texts, they become acquainted with new attitudes and values, new ways of thinking about themselves, new ways of thinking about others, and new possibilities for acting in the world. Once practitioners absorb these possibilities, they begin to develop intentions for implementing them in everyday experience, and to develop specific plans for executing them.

Other Buddhist traditions change conduct through Metta practices (e.g. Kornbloom, 2008; Salzberg, 2011). During these practices, meditators generate constructive emotions – such as loving kindness and compassion – towards a diverse collection of other people, including individuals for whom they might normally experience intense negative emotion. By generating these emotions towards others on a regular basis, practitioners establish these new mental habits in memory that change their perceptions of people and their actions toward them. In important ways, Lojong and Metta practices are much like Cognitive Behavioural Therapies that aim to develop new knowledge structures, automatic responses, and behaviours (e.g. Beck & Dozois, 2011; Hayes, 2004).

From the dual-process perspective, Lojong and Metta practices present guidelines, instructions, and examples for practitioners that implement long-term behavioural change via a wide variety of regulatory activities. Initially, RRs absorb and implement the teachings. Ultimately, however, these RRs establish new IRs that come to dominate thought, emotion, and action (as increasingly demonstrated by empirical research; e.g. Hofmann, Grossman, & Hinton, 2011). Again, the dual-process perspective offers a useful framework for understanding the regulatory processes that initiate and eventually produce these long-term changes. The large theoretical and empirical literatures on creating meaning, developing new narratives, and redirecting goals offer useful perspectives on how conduct practices operate (e.g. Pennebaker, 1997; Stanovich et al., 2014; Wilson, 2011). Conversely, conduct practices are likely to offer new insights into similar Western interventions.

To the extent that conduct practices are successful, they lead to positive social qualities such as the *Brahmaviharas*, which include loving kindness, compassion, sympathetic joy, and equanimity (e.g. Wallace, 1999). Because conduct practices also diminish self-absorption, the related processes of destructive emotion and mind-wandering become less likely, as do grasping and aversion. As self-related thoughts become less prevalent, equanimity follows, as does becoming more present in the world. When actions are performed, they are less likely to be self-serving and more likely to serve the general good and the needs of others.

Wisdom practices

Once mindfulness, equanimity, and ethical conduct have been established, some of the more advanced Buddhist practices become possible (e.g. Namgyal, 2001; Norbu, 1983; Schmidt, 2004; Thrangu, 2004). The aims of these practices include understanding the nature of mind and becoming increasingly liberated from samsara.

Once the ability to focus attention has become free from mind-wandering and other self-absorbed distractions, the practitioner can focus on conscious experience, both introspective and perceptual. As various aspects of consciousness receive attention, they are examined to better understand their nature. For example, each aspect of consciousness is assessed for whether it is real or simply a construction of the mind. Ultimately, the goal is to see that every aspect of consciousness is an impermanent conditioned construction that arises and dissipates. Although this is obvious for dreams and illusions, it is less obvious for thoughts and perceptions, which typically seem real. Also targeted by this practice is the idea that perceived entities and events have essences, reflecting some kind of true nature in reality. Again, the goal is to see that these essences don't actually exist and are simply constructions of mind.

Although all aspects of consciousness are examined in this manner, conscious experiences of the self and the external world are of particular importance. To increasingly reduce the grasping and aversion associated with pursuing self-interest, wisdom practices help the pratitioner see the self as a conditioned construction with forms that arise and dissipate in experience. Once this realization occurs, the force of self on thought, emotion, and action decreases. Analogously, to understand the nature of perception, wisdom practices help the practitioner see through the compelling (and important) illusion that perceived states exist externally (e.g. as in vision). Instead, perceptions are internal constructions that don't really exist outside the person as they appear, but belong to a general field of consciousness within the mind. Once the true natures of self-perception and external perception are perceived, they no longer carry the significance they once did. As their psychological natures become increasingly understood, they decreasingly initiate the constant grasping and aversion that underlie samsara.

As wisdom practices make the nature of consciousness increasingly apparent, the normal dualism of experience increasingly dissipates into a non-dual state during contemplative practice (e.g. Dunne, 2015). Rather than experiencing fundamental distinctions between the self and the external world, or of the self acting on objects, these distinctions increasingly collapse in consciousness. Practitioners enter the *natural state*, where consciousness exists without a sense of a self evaluating and acting in an external world, without a sense of lack or imbalance (e.g. Namgyal, 2001; Norbu, 1983; Schmidt, 2004; Thrangu, 2004). Consciousness simply exists, less obscured by the conditioning that underlies samsara. While in these states, a practitioner may still act, think, and feel emotion, as the causal structures established in conduct practices produce ethical conduct (e.g. Dunne, 2015). There is much less sense, however, of a self acting, thinking, and feeling.

Many practitioners may not perform practices aimed at producing non-dual states or aspire to experience them. Nevertheless, wisdom practices stand as a testament to what's possible with disciplined regulatory processing. Once mindfulness and conduct practices diminish problems associated with IRs, wisdom practices focus on understanding the nature of mind, further dissolving the illusions that contribute to samsara. By developing RRs that examine the nature of consciousness, it becomes possible to attain critical insights about how the mind works.

RRs developed during wisdom practices complement other RRs developed during earlier practices along the Eight-Fold Path. Together, all these RRs constitute an extensive regulatory system that not only regulates experience in the moment, but that also changes behaviour, emotion, and thought in the long term, with newly created IRs fundamentally changing how a person thinks, feels, and acts. From the dual-process perspective, this regulatory system has tamed the 10,000-pound gorilla responsible for the constant barrage of dysfunctional IRs that underlie samsara.

Discussion

I began with the observation that dual-process theories have been applied extensively to cognitive and social phenomena for more than 100 years. This chapter has similarly attempted to apply dual-process theories to contemplative practices that have existed for thousands of years in Buddhism. As we have seen, a striking rapport exists between them.

Most basically, the two kinds of processes central in dual-process theories – IRs and RRs – are readily apparent throughout Buddhism. On the one hand, IRs underlie the dissatisfaction and unhappiness that Buddhism aims to address, which are produced by the root causes of self-illusion, grasping, and aversion. On the other hand, an impressive system of RRs constituting the Eight-Fold Path offer a means of transforming dissatisfaction and unhappiness, creating healthier IRs in the process. Because dual-process theories map so well onto Buddhism, the large bodies of theory and research associated with these theories can be brought to bear on informing its basic principles, such as The Four Noble Truths, karma, samsara, and mindfulness.

Conversely, Buddhism offers considerable potential for better understanding dual-process theories. As we saw earlier, the root causes of samsara – grasping, aversion, and self-relevance – provide insights into the causes of the unhappiness, psychopathology, and other dysfunctional aspects of the human condition. Similarly, the integrated approach of the Eight-Fold Path, together with its individual practices, offers ideas for regulatory interventions that could be adapted effectively in Western contexts, and that already have been to a considerable extent (e.g. mindfulness and compassion practices). An intriguing possibility is that integrated collections of interventions could be developed in the Western tradition that are analogous to the Eight-Fold Path in Buddhism.

Perhaps the most gains to be made will result from integrating the two approaches in areas where doing so is relevant. When developing social and clinical interventions that have a contemplative character, for example, drawing on both explanatory frameworks and integrating their relevant insights may offer the greatest opportunity for success. Whereas the Western framework excels at working with unconscious cognitive and neural mechanisms, the Buddhist framework excels at working with conscious experience and daily practice. Although both have converged on remarkably similar accounts of the mind in many ways (as reflected in the common importance of IRs and RRs), they nevertheless offer complementary accounts of the same phenomena, each providing unique insights.

As researchers work increasingly with both frameworks together, a likely outcome is that each explanatory framework will have significant influence on the other, such that hybrids emerge. Based on what we have seen, much potential for mutual influence exists: first, in understanding the causal systems of IRs that dominate behaviour, emotion, and thought; and second, in developing sophisticated systems of RRs that manage IRs in the moment and change them in the long term.

Author notes

The ideas in this chapter were presented in a talk to the Mind and Life Summer Research Institute in June 2014. I am grateful to John Dunne, Johan Karremans, and Esther Papies for helpful comments on an earlier draft. Any errors that remain are my sole responsibility. Address correspondence to Lawrence W. Barsalou, Institute of Neuroscience and Psychology, 58 Hillhead Street, University of Glasgow, Glasgow G12 8QB UK, lawrence.barsalou@glasgow.ac.uk, http://barsaloulab.org.

Notes

1 So that the acronyms to follow will be easily decodable, I only use IR for *Initial Responses* and RR for *Regulatory Responses* (instead of IIR for *Involuntary Initial Responses* and ORR for *Optional Regulatory Responses*). Nevertheless, the assumption remains that initial

responses tend to be *involuntary*, reflecting the bottom-up activation of modality-specific pathways, whereas regulatory responses tend to be *optional*, primarily occurring when sufficient motivation, capacity, and knowledge exist.

2 Although I focus on the bottom-up activation of IRs here, it is essential to note that these activations operate in the context of extensive top-down processing (e.g. Barsalou, 2009, 2016; Clark, 2013; Friston, 2010; McClelland & Rumelhart, 1981). Background processing typically produces top-down predictions about objects and events likely to be encountered in the current situation, together with extensive top-down inferences about them once they occur.

References

Baird, B., Smallwood, J., & Schooler, J. W. (2011). Back to the future: Autobiographical planning and the functionality of mind-wandering. *Consciousness and Cognition, 20,* 1604–1611.

Barrett, L. F., & Bliss-Moreau, E. (2009). Affect as a psychological primitive. *Advances in Experimental Social Psychology, 41,* 167–218.

Barsalou, L. W. (2009). Simulation, situated conceptualization, and prediction. *Philosophical Transactions of the Royal Society B: Biological Sciences, 364,* 1281–1289.

Barsalou, L. W. (2016). Situated conceptualization: Theory and applications. In Y. Coello & M. H. Fischer (Eds.), *Foundations of embodied cognition* (pp. 11–37). East Sussex: Psychology Press.

Baumeister, R. F. (1998). The self. In D. T. Gilbert, S. T. Fiske, & G. Lindzey (Eds.), *The handbook of social psychology* (4th ed., Vols. 1 and 2, pp. 680–740). New York: McGraw-Hill.

Beck, A. T., & Dozois, D. J. A. (2011). Cognitive therapy: Current status and future directions. *Annual Review of Medicine, 62,* 397–409.

Berger, A. (2011). *Self-regulation: Brain, cognition, and development* (Vol. XIV). Washington, DC: American Psychological Association.

Bishop, S. R., Lau, M., Shapiro, S., Carlson, L., Anderson, N. D., Carmody, J., . . . Devins, G. (2006). Mindfulness: A proposed operational definition. *Clinical Psychology: Science and Practice, 11,* 230–241.

Bodhi, B. (2005). *In the Buddha's words.* Boston: Wisdom Publications.

Buckner, R. L., & Krienen, F. M. (2013). The evolution of distributed association networks in the human brain. *Trends in Cognitive Sciences, 17,* 648–665.

Chaiken, S., & Trope, Y. (1999). *Dual-process theories in social psychology.* New York: Guilford Press.

Chaumon, M., Kveraga, K., Barrett, L. F., & Bar, M. (2014). Visual predictions in the orbitofrontal cortex rely on associative content. *Cerebral Cortex, 24,* 2899–2907.

Chun, M. M., Golomb, J. D., & Turk-Browne, N. B. (2011). A taxonomy of external and internal attention. *Annual Review of Psychology, 62,* 73–101.

Clark, A. (2013). Whatever next? Predictive brains, situated agents, and the future of cognitive science. *Behavioral and Brain Sciences, 36,* 1–73.

Dahl, C. J., Lutz, A., & Davidson, R. J. (2015). Reconstructing and deconstructing the self: Cognitive mechanisms in meditation practice. *Trends in Cognitive Sciences, 19,* 515–523.

Dickenson, J., Berkman, E. T., Arch, J., & Lieberman, M. D. (2013). Neural correlates of focused attention during a brief mindfulness induction. *Social Cognitive and Affective Neuroscience, 8,* 40–47.

Dreyfus, G. (2008). An Abhidharmic view of emotional pathologies and their remedies. In A. Harrington & A. Zajonc (Eds.), *The Dalai Lama at MIT* (pp. 122–135). Cambridge, MA: Harvard University Press.

Dreyfus, G. (2011). Is mindfulness present-centred and non-judgemental? A discussion of the cognitive dimensions of mindfulness. *Contemporary Buddhism, 12,* 41–54.

Dunne, J. D. (2011). Toward an understanding of non-dual mindfulness. *Contemporary Buddhism, 12,* 71–88.

Dunne, J. D. (2015). Buddhist styles of mindfulness: A heuristic approach. In B. D. Ostafin, M. D. Robinson, & B. P. Meier (Eds.), *Handbook of mindfulness and self-regulation* (pp. 251–270). New York: Springer.

Evans, J. S. B. T. (1984). Heuristic and analytic processes in reasoning. *British Journal of Psychology, 75,* 451–468.

Frable, D. E. (1997). Gender, racial, ethnic, sexual, and class identities. *Annual Review of Psychology, 48,* 139–162.

Friston, K. (2010). The free-energy principle: A unified brain theory? *Nature Reviews Neuroscience, 11,* 127–138.

Fronsdal, G. (2001). *The issue at hand.* Barry, MA: Insight Meditation Center.

Gawronski, B., & Payne, B. K. (2011). *Handbook of implicit social cognition: Measurement, theory, and applications.* New York: Guilford Press.

Gerlach, K. D., Spreng, R. N., Madore, K. P., & Schacter, D. L. (2014). Future planning: Default network activity couples with frontoparietal control network and reward-processing regions during process and outcome simulations. *Social Cognitive and Affective Neuroscience, 9,* 1942–1951.

Gethin, R. (2010). *The foundations of Buddhism.* Oxford: Oxford University Press.

Goleman, D. (2003). *Destructive emotions: How we can overcome them: A scientific dialogue with the Dalai Lama.* New York: Bantam Books.

Goschke, T. (2013). Volition in action: Intentions, control dilemmas and the dynamic regulation of intentional control. In W. Prinz, M. Beisert, & A. Herwig (Eds.), *Action science: Foundations of an emerging discipline* (pp. 409–434). Cambridge, MA: MIT Press.

Greenwald, A. G., & Banaji, M. R. (1995). Implicit social cognition: Attitudes, self-esteem, and stereotypes. *Psychological Review, 102,* 4–27.

Hasenkamp, W., Wilson-Mendenhall, C. D., Duncan, E., & Barsalou, L. W. (2012). Mind-wandering and attention during focused meditation: A fine-grained temporal analysis of fluctuating cognitive states. *NeuroImage, 59,* 750–760.

Hayes, S. C. (2004). Acceptance and commitment therapy, relational frame theory, and the third wave of behavioral and cognitive therapies. *Behavior Therapy, 35,* 639–665.

Hermans, D., De Houwer, J., & Eelen, P. (2001). A time course analysis of the affective priming effect. *Cognition & Emotion, 15,* 143–165.

Herring, D. R., White, K. R., Jabeen, L. N., Hinojos, M., Terrazas, G., Reyes, S. M., . . . Crites, S. L. (2013). On the automatic activation of attitudes: A quarter century of evaluative priming research. *Psychological Bulletin, 139,* 1062–1089.

Hofmann, S. G., Grossman, P., & Hinton, D. E. (2011). Loving-kindness and compassion meditation: Potential for psychological interventions. *Clinical Psychology Review, 31,* 1126–1132.

Hofmann, W., Baumeister, R. F., Förster, G., & Vohs, K. D. (2012). Everyday temptations: An experience sampling study of desire, conflict, and self-control. *Journal of Personality and Social Psychology, 102,* 1318–1335.

Hofmann, W., Schmeichel, B. J., & Baddeley, A. D. (2012). Executive functions and self-regulation. *Trends in Cognitive Sciences, 16,* 174–180.

James, W. (1890/1950). *The principles of psychology.* New York: Dover.

Jinpa, T. (2006). *Mind training: The great collection.* Somerville, MA: Wisdom Publications.

Kabat-Zinn, J. (1994). *Wherever you go, there you are: Mindfulness meditation in everyday life.* New York: Hyperion Books.

Kane, M. J., & McVay, J. C. (2012). What mind-wandering reveals about executive-control abilities and failures. *Current Directions in Psychological Science, 21*, 348–354.

Kavanagh, D. J., Andrade, J., & May, J. (2005). Imaginary relish and exquisite torture: The elaborated intrusion theory of desire. *Psychological Review, 112*, 446–467.

Killingsworth, M. A., & Gilbert, D. T. (2010). A wandering mind is an unhappy mind. *Science, 330*, 932–932.

King, S. B. (2009). *Socially engaged Buddhism.* Honolulu: University of Hawaii Press.

Kornbloom, J. (2008). *Meditation for beginners.* Louisville, CO: Sounds True.

Kucyi, A., & Davis, K. D. (2014). Dynamic functional connectivity of the default mode network tracks daydreaming. *NeuroImage, 100*, 471–480.

Lahey, B. B. (2009). Public health significance of neuroticism. *American Psychologist, 64*, 241–256.

Lebois, L. A. M., Papies, E. K., Gopinath, K., Cabanban, R., Quigley, K. S., Krishnamurthy, V., . . . Barsalou, L. W. (2015). A shift in perspective: Decentering through mindful attention to imagined stressful events. *Neuropsychologia, 75*, 505–524.

Lebrecht, S., Bar, M., Barrett, L. F., & Tarr, M. J. (2012). Micro-valences: Perceiving affective valence in everyday objects. *Frontiers in Psychology, 3*, 107.

Loy, D. R. (2002). *A Buddhist history of the West: Studies in lack.* New York: SUNY Press.

Lutz, A., Jha, A. P., Dunne, J. D., & Saron, C. D. (2015). Investigating the phenomenological matrix of mindfulness-related practices from a neurocognitive perspective. *American Psychologist, 70*, 632–658.

Markus, H., & Wurf, E. (1987). The dynamic self-concept: A social psychological perspective. *Annual Review of Psychology, 38*, 299–337.

McClelland, J. L., & Rumelhart, D. E. (1981). An interactive activation model of context effects in letter perception: I. An account of basic findings. *Psychological Review, 88*, 375–407.

Metcalfe, J., & Mischel, W. (1999). A hot/cool-system analysis of delay of gratification: Dynamics of willpower. *Psychological Review, 106*(1), 3–19.

Mischel, W., Ayduk, O., Berman, M. G., Casey, B. J., Gotlib, I. H., Jonides, J., . . . Shoda, Y. (2011). 'Willpower' over the life span: Decomposing self-regulation. *Social Cognitive and Affective Neuroscience, 6*, 252–256.

Mittner, M., Boekel, W., Tucker, A. M., Turner, B. M., Heathcote, A., & Forstmann, B. U. (2014). When the brain takes a break: A model-based analysis of mind-wandering. *The Journal of Neuroscience, 34*, 16286–16295.

Moors, A., & De Houwer, J. (2006). Automaticity: A theoretical and conceptual analysis. *Psychological Bulletin, 132*, 297–326.

Mrazek, M. D., Smallwood, J., Franklin, M. S., Chin, J. M., Baird, B., & Schooler, J. W. (2012). The role of mind-wandering in measurements of general aptitude. *Journal of Experimental Psychology: General, 141*, 788–798.

Namgyal, D. T. (2001). *Clarifying the natural state.* Nepal: Rangjung Yeshe Publications.

Norbu, N. (1983). *The mirror: Advice on the presence of awareness.* Barrytown, NY: Barrytown.

Northoff, G., Heinzel, A., de Greck, M., Bermpohl, F., Dobrowolny, H., & Panksepp, J. (2006). Self-referential processing in our brain – A meta-analysis of imaging studies on the self. *NeuroImage, 31*, 440–457.

Papies, E. K., & Barsalou, L. W. (2015). Grounding desire and motivated behavior: A theoretical framework and review of empirical evidence. In W. Hofmann & L. F. Nordgren (Eds.), *The psychology of desire* (pp. 36–60). New York: Guilford Press.

Papies, E. K., Barsalou, L. W., & Custers, R. (2012). Mindful attention prevents mindless impulses. *Social Psychological and Personality Science, 3*, 291–299.

Papies, E. K., Pronk, T. M., Keesman, M., & Barsalou, L. W. (2015). The benefits of simply observing: Mindful attention modulates the link between motivation and behavior. *Journal of Personality and Social Psychology, 108*, 148–170.

Pennebaker, J. W. (1997). *Opening up: The healing power of expressing emotions*. New York: Guilford.

Posner, M. I., & Snyder, C. R. R. (1975). Attention and cognitive control. In R. L. Solso (Ed.), *Information processing and cognition* (pp. 205–223). Hillsdale, NJ: Lawrence Erlbaum.

Qin, P., & Northoff, G. (2011). How is our self related to midline regions and the default-mode network? *NeuroImage, 57*, 1221–1233.

Ricard, M. (2007). *Happiness: A guide to developing life's most important skill*. London: Atlantic.

Rudebeck, P. H., & Murray, E. A. (2014). The orbitofrontal oracle: Cortical mechanisms for the prediction and evaluation of specific behavioral outcomes. *Neuron, 84*, 1143–1156.

Salzberg, S. (2011). *Real happiness: The power of meditation*. New York: Workman.

Schmidt, M. B. (2004). *Dzogchen essentials*. Kathmandu: Rangjung Yeshe Publications.

Schneider, W., & Shiffrin, R. M. (1977). Controlled and automatic human information processing: I. Detection, search, and attention. *Psychological Review, 84*, 1–66.

Sharma, L., Markon, K. E., & Clark, L. A. (2014). Toward a theory of distinct types of 'impulsive' behaviors: A meta-analysis of self-report and behavioral measures. *Psychological Bulletin, 140*, 374–408.

Sheline, Y. I., Barch, D. M., Price, J. L., Rundle, M. M., Vaishnavi, S. N., Snyder, A. Z., . . . Raichle, M. E. (2009). The default mode network and self-referential processes in depression. *Proceedings of the National Academy of Sciences, 106*, 1942–1947.

Shenhav, A., Barrett, L. F., & Bar, M. (2012). Affective value and associative processing share a cortical substrate. *Cognitive, Affective, & Behavioral Neuroscience, 13*, 46–59.

Sherman, J. W., Gawronski, B., & Trope, Y. (2014). *Dual-process theories of the social mind*. New York: Guilford Publications.

Sloman, S. A. (1996). The empirical case for two systems of reasoning. *Psychological Bulletin, 119*, 3–22.

Stahl, C., Voss, A., Schmitz, F., Nuszbaum, M., Tüscher, O., Lieb, K., & Klauer, K. C. (2014). Behavioral components of impulsivity. *Journal of Experimental Psychology: General, 143*, 850–866.

Stanovich, K. E., & West, R. F. (2000). Individual differences in reasoning: Implications for the rationality debate. *Behavioral and Brain Sciences, 23*, 645–665.

Stanovich, K. E., West, R. F., & Toplak, M. E. (2014). Rationality, intelligence, and the defining features of Type 1 and Type 2 processing. In J. W. Sherman, B. Gawronski, & Y. Trope (Eds.), *Dual-process theories of the social mind* (pp. 386–399). New York: Guilford.

Strack, F., & Deutsch, R. (2004). Reflective and impulsive determinants of social behavior. *Personality and Social Psychology Review, 8*, 220–247.

Sui, J., & Humphreys, G. W. (2015a). More of me! Distinguishing self and reward bias using redundancy gains. *Attention, Perception & Psychophysics, 77*, 2549–2561.

Sui, J., & Humphreys, G. W. (2015b). Super-size me: Self biases increase to larger stimuli. *Psychonomic Bulletin & Review, 22*, 550–558.

Sui, J., Liu, M., Mevorach, C., & Humphreys, G. W. (2015). The salient self: The left intraparietal sulcus responds to social as well as perceptual-salience after self-association. *Cerebral Cortex, 25*, 1060–1068.

Sui, J., Rotshtein, P., & Humphreys, G. W. (2013). Coupling social attention to the self forms a network for personal significance. *Proceedings of the National Academy of Sciences, 110*, 7607–7612.

Thompson, D. R., Besner, D., & Smilek, D. (2015). A resource-control account of sustained attention: Evidence from mind-wandering and vigilance paradigms. *Perspectives on Psychological Science, 10*, 82–96.

Thrangu, K. (2004). *Essentials of Mahamudra: Looking directly at the mind*. Somerville, MA: Wisdom Publications.

Tincher, M. M., Lebois, L. A. M., & Barsalou, L. W. (2015). Mindful attention reduces linguistic intergroup bias. *Mindfulness, 7,* 349–360.

Wallace, B. A. (1999). *The four immeasurables: Practices to open the heart.* Ithaca, NY: Snow Lion.

Wilson, R. C., Takahashi, Y. K., Schoenbaum, G., & Niv, Y. (2014). Orbitofrontal cortex as a cognitive map of task space. *Neuron, 81,* 267–279.

Wilson, T. D. (2004). *Strangers to ourselves.* Cambridge, MA: Harvard University Press.

Wilson, T. D. (2011). *Redirect: The surprising new science of psychological change.* London: Penguin.

Winkielman, P., Berridge, K. C., & Wilbarger, J. L. (2005). Unconscious affective reactions to masked happy versus angry faces influence consumption behavior and judgements of value. *Personality and Social Psychology Bulletin, 31,* 121–135.

4

THE HYPO-EGOIC IMPACT OF MINDFULNESS ON SELF, IDENTITY, AND THE PROCESSING OF SELF-RELEVANT INFORMATION

Mark R. Leary and Kate J. Diebels

Most people who are familiar with mindfulness, whether through knowledge of the scholarly literature or personal experience, recognize that mindfulness has interesting and important implications for an array of psychological and interpersonal outcomes. People who score high on trait-like measures of mindfulness fare better emotionally, have more positive interpersonal relationships, and display greater general well-being than people who score lower, and interventions designed to enhance mindfulness lead to improvements in emotional well-being, resilience, relationships, and physical health (Brown, Creswell, & Ryan, 2015). Fundamentally, mindfulness is a cognitive-attentional habit that, like all habits, can be strengthened through practice. Thus, over time, continued practice of mindfulness causes people to become more dispositionally mindful (Kiken, Garland, Bluth, Paisson, & Gaylord, 2015).

Yet, despite strong evidence that mindfulness is psychologically beneficial, relatively little attention has been devoted to the precise nature of the psychological processes that underlie individual differences in trait mindfulness and the psychological mediators of mindfulness training. Certainly, we know a great deal about downstream consequences of mindfulness, but what are the fundamental psychological processes that underlie these effects?

Our goal in this chapter is to provide an overarching perspective on the nature and mechanisms of mindfulness based on theory and research dealing with self-awareness, identity, and self-relevant thought. Although traditional perspectives on mindfulness stressed the role of mindfulness in remediating problems created by the "self" (Boisselier, 1993; Epstein, 1995), surprisingly little psychological work has focused explicitly on the effects of mindfulness on self and identity (see, however, Hölzel, Lazar, Gard, Schuman-Olivier, Vago, & Ott, 2011). The gist of our analysis is that, at its foundation, mindfulness involves ways of processing self-relevant information that differ from how people typically think about themselves when not being mindful, and that these processing differences are responsible for many, if not most, of the effects of mindfulness. We do not claim that our analysis necessarily captures all of the relevant mechanisms of action, but we do assert that, at its core, mindfulness involves a distinct way of thinking about oneself.

Self-awareness and egoic thought

The most familiar definition of mindfulness is Kabat-Zinn's (1994) claim that mindfulness involves "paying attention in a particular way: on purpose, in the present moment, and nonjudgmentally" (p. 4), a view echoed by Bishop et al.'s (2004) conceptualization of mindfulness as "a kind of nonelaborative, nonjudgmental, present centered awareness" (p. 232). But why does intentionally paying non-judgemental attention in the present moment create the outcomes that are associated with mindfulness?

To answer this question requires that we consider the nature of human self-awareness. Although we do not know for certain when our prehuman ancestors acquired the ability to think consciously about themselves (Leary & Buttermore, 2003), before the evolution of self-awareness, hominids would have been naturally and inherently "mindful," to use the term loosely. Without the ability to think consciously, they would have been chronically attentive to stimuli in their immediate environment, as well as to their internal sensations, which they would have experienced without cognitive elaboration, internal commentary, or judgement. Like other species that lack the capacity to self-reflect, our prehuman ancestors would have experienced the world as it unfolded before them, but, not having the capacity for complex, self-relevant thought, they could not have "talked to themselves" about what they were experiencing.

Nor would they have been able to imagine themselves in other places and times or anticipated, planned for, or worried about future events. (Perhaps they were able to look a few minutes ahead, as chimpanzees and bonobos appear to do [Mulcahy & Call, 2006], but they could not have undertaken long-term plans.) Without self-awareness, they also would not have consciously evaluated themselves, compared themselves to other people, or sought ways to improve themselves. And, although they would have experienced fear and other negative emotions when threatening events arose, they would not have created negative emotions through self-thought when external conditions were OK at the moment.

When and why self-awareness arose is unclear (Leary & Buttermore, 2003), but it provided many advantages that set human beings on a unique path as a species. Being able to think consciously about themselves allowed human beings to learn from their past actions and plan consciously for the future. They could also use mental analogues of themselves much like computer avatars to simulate alternate courses of action in their minds (Leary, Estrada, & Allen, 2009). Self-awareness also allowed people to think about who they were and what they were like, providing self-views that guided their actions. Self-awareness also led people to think about what other people might be thinking about them, which helped them navigate social life but also made them worry about how they were viewed by others (Leary, 2004).

Each of these features of self-awareness was immensely beneficial, and it is hard to imagine the state of humanity today if people could not plan, introspect, self-evaluate, and consider other people's views of them. This capacity led human beings to dominate most other life forms on earth and paved the way for the defining features of human civilizations, such as philosophy, religion, science, politics, business, medicine, and education, all of which require conscious self-reflection.

Yet self-awareness came with a downside: It pulled people's attention away from their immediate experience to an inner world of self-relevant thought. To be sure, some of those thoughts were beneficial in dealing with life, but many of them were not. Once people became self-aware – and particularly after the agricultural revolution moved them from the present-focused lifestyle of hunters and gatherers to the future-focused lifestyle of agriculturalists (Martin, 1999) – people began to tend to think about themselves more frequently than needed to deal effectively with the demands of everyday living. They began to engage in an incessant stream of self-talk as they ruminated about past events, planned for and worried about events that might occur in the future, and incessantly thought about their personal concerns. Despite its extensive advantages, self-awareness often created a self-generated hell of excessive self-preoccupation (Baumeister, 1991; Leary, 2004).

In addition to contributing to excessive self-awareness and concern about the future, self-reflection seems to have compounded people's natural level of self-interest. All animals are self-interested in the sense that they look after their own (and sometimes their kin's) concerns and protect the resources needed for survival and reproduction. But one does not get the sense that other animals spend time thinking about their personal interests when they are not actively pursuing them. Yet, because they are self-aware, human beings think a great deal about what they want (and how to get more of it) – not only material provisions but also symbolic outcomes. Despite the self-regulatory capacity that self-awareness affords (Duval & Wicklund, 1972), it seems to have led human beings to become more selfish and egoistic than any other animal.

The hypo-egoic nature of mindfulness

Many sages, philosophers, spiritual teachers, and psychologists have recognized the pernicious effects of egoic self-thought. Gautama Buddha, the sage whose teachings stimulated what became known as Buddhism, was among the first to articulate these problems clearly and fully, pointing out that people's self-thoughts are a major determinant of their dissatisfaction and suffering. He also advocated an approach to training one's mind in a way that changes self-relevant thought and provided the basis for many schools of meditation and for the practice of mindfulness. (In many ways, Buddha could be regarded as the first cognitive therapist.) Viewed through the lens of contemporary views of self-awareness, mindfulness reduces many of the problems that arose from the emergence of self-awareness.

Mindfulness has its effects, we believe, by promoting a style of thinking – a mindset – in which people's self-relevant thoughts are fewer, more present-focused, more concrete, less introspective, and less evaluative than they typically are. We call this mindset "hypo-egoic" to reflect the fact that its central feature is a lower-than-normal level of self-preoccupation. People operating in a hypo-egoic mindset are less self-focused, self-preoccupied, and ego-involved than they are in the typical egoic mindset in which they usually operate (Leary & Diebels, 2013; Leary & Terry, 2012). Although hypo-egoic states can arise spontaneously (as when people are in flow, experience awe, or have a mystical experience [see Brown & Leary, 2016]), people often take intentional steps to induce hypo-egoic states. Practicing mindfulness and other forms of meditation are among the most tried-and-true approaches for promoting hypo-egoicism. To be clear, mindfulness does not eliminate self-awareness or make people "self-less." Rather, it changes the amount and nature of self-attention and self-thought to be less self-focused and self-interested than it typically is. And, in so doing, it reduces the problems that arose when human beings became self-aware. But how does it do that? What processes are involved?

First, mindfulness inherently involves heightened attention to the present situation and one's reactions to it, and, conversely, fewer thoughts about the past and future. (Indeed, all conceptualizations and measures of mindfulness concur that a person who is oblivious to the present moment and caught up in thoughts about past or future is certainly not being mindful.) But what does this present focus entail? Is it better viewed as concentrated attention on the present moment that leaves few cognitive resources for problematic self-relevant thoughts, or as a diminution of self-relevant thinking, which frees cognitive resources to allow more prolonged attention to the present moment? Mindfulness training typically emphasizes both of these processes, encouraging people to attend to current sights, sounds, and sensations while letting thoughts pass through the mind without elaboration or judgement. In either case, mindfulness involves a reduction in self-relevant thoughts about the past and present, which attenuates many of the problems associated with excessive self-relevant thought and egoism.

Second, when engaged in mindfulness, people tend to think about concrete rather than abstract aspects of themselves and their behaviour, another central feature of hypo-egoic mindsets (Leary & Diebels, 2013). Contrary to the popular belief that mindfulness involves pressing the self's mute button to stop all thoughts, mindful people may, in fact, attend to and think about what they are doing. But they do so in a concrete fashion with no more internal commentary or abstraction than is needed to do whatever the present situation requires. Research shows that mindfulness is associated with concrete processing (Watkins, 2015). Thinking about oneself in a concrete fashion virtually eliminates egoic concerns, which are symbolically mediated and usually involve thinking about the future implications of whatever is happening. Concrete self-thoughts also minimize the degree to which evaluations of oneself in the present situation – which are needed to gauge the effectiveness of one's ongoing behaviour – are generalized to judgements of oneself overall. For example, people may evaluate what they are doing at the moment for purposes of completing a task without generalizing those evaluations of concrete behaviours to abstract evaluations of their ability or other characteristics.

The present-focused attention and concrete self-thoughts that characterize hypo-egoic states, including mindfulness, are inextricably linked. Abstract and symbolic self-thoughts require that people draw upon abstract information involving previous experiences, symbolic self-views, or implicational thinking about the future. In contrast, whatever one is doing in the present moment is usually highly concrete and specific.

Third, like other states that involve a hypo-egoic mindset, mindfulness involves minimal introspection. Although people in a mindful state are aware of their thoughts and subjective experiences (sometimes acutely so), they do not mull over their thoughts, feelings, or motives or ruminate about themselves except as needed to act in the present moment.

Finally, mindfulness involves a non-judgemental attitude toward oneself and whatever is happening. In the typical egoic mindset, people chronically judge events that occur with respect to their personal concerns (Kiken & Shook, 2011), and these judgements often evoke emotional reactions. In a mindful state, such judgements are minimal, arising only when needed for immediate action.

Hypo-egoic manifestations of mindfulness

Our thesis is that many, if not most, of the cognitive, emotional, and behavioural features of mindfulness can be traced to the fact that it is a hypo-egoic state in which people's self-relevant thoughts tend to be fewer, present-focused, concrete, non-introspective, and relatively non-evaluative. In this section, we explore the role of hypo-egoic mindsets in the relationship between mindfulness and people's self-construals, values, reactions to undesired events, defensiveness, and social relationships.

Self-construals

As people observe themselves with mindful, non-judgemental attention, they think about themselves differently than they do in an egoic state. For starters, evidence suggests that mindfulness helps people to have more accurate views of themselves by counteracting both informational and motivational barriers to accurate self-knowledge (Carlson, 2013). Specifically, purposeful self-directed attention, without interpretation or internal commentary, may increase the amount of objective information that people have about themselves. In addition, observing oneself non-evaluatively may reduce self-serving biases that spring from self-enhancement and ego-defensiveness (Carlson, 2013; Wayment, Bauer, & Sylaska, 2014).

Along these lines, people who score higher in trait mindfulness have a clearer, more discriminating understanding of their own emotions (Brewer, Elwafi, & Davis, 2013; Hill & Updegraff, 2012), and mindfulness leads people who are depressed to recall aversive memories in greater detail (Hargus, Crane, Barnhofer, & Williams, 2010). Mindful people are also more accurate in predicting how they will be affected by future events (Emanuel, Updegraff, Kalmbach, & Ciesla, 2010).

Mindfulness may also influence self-construals by leading people to distinguish more clearly between who they are, and their thoughts and images of who they are. A common theme in mindfulness training is that thoughts are not reality and, thus, need not be taken too seriously (Lebois et al., 2015; Papies, Pronk, Keesman, & Barsalou, 2015; Ryan & Rigby, 2015). When applied to oneself, this perspective may diminish the importance that people place on both their views of themselves and other people's views of them (Brown, Ryan, Creswell, & Niemiec, 2008). Of course, self-views and social images sometimes have meaningful implications and, thus, require attention and care. Yet, to the extent that mindfulness helps people recognize the ephemeral nature of thoughts, people may become less invested in their own self-views.

Third, hypo-egoic states are often associated with changes in people's views of themselves. As mindful people observe the ever-changing flux of sensations and perceptions that make up their experience in any given moment, they may start seeing themselves more as a "dynamic process, a shifting web of relations among evanescent aspects of [themselves] such as perceptions, ideas, and desires" (Galin, 2003, p. 108) than as either a fixed physical entity or a homunculus-type "thing" at the centre of their experiences.

As they begin to observe mindfully how events and other people affect them, they may come to realize their interdependence with their environment, bolstering the sense of interconnection between themselves and the external world. Rather than seeing themselves as separate and *apart from* other people and the world, they begin to see themselves as *a part of* the groups, communities, and greater whole in which they're embedded. And the more connected they feel, the more they include other people and even the natural world into their identity (Leary, Tipsord, & Tate, 2008).

Values

Values reflect standards for evaluating events and goals that motivate action. Schwartz (1994) identified 10 universal values that can be grouped according to two dimensions. For our purposes, one of those dimensions – self-enhancement versus self-transcendence – is of interest because, in fostering hypo-egoism, mindfulness should be associated with changes in the importance that people place on these values. A reduction of egoic thought, with its excessive self-preoccupation, should result in lower prioritization of values associated with self-enhancement (which emphasize pursuing one's own interests via success and power) and greater emphasis on self-transcendence values (which emphasize concern for the interests and welfare of others). (Technically, "self-transcendence" is a misnomer in this context because people are not transcending themselves as much as they are simply less self-preoccupied and self-interested.) The less that people are preoccupied with their own concerns, the more attuned they can be to other people and the larger world (Farb et al., 2007; Parker, Nelson, Epel, & Siegel, 2015; Phelan, 2010). Thus, hypo-egoic states, including mindfulness, should be associated with a tendency to prioritize self-transcendent values such as benevolence (maintaining and enhancing the welfare of people with whom one is in frequent personal contact – that is, one's in-group) and universalism (appreciating and protecting all people, animals, and the natural world).

The goals that modern Western society tends to value and promote – such as autonomy, status, power, self-promotion, and success – tend to be self-focused, and evidence suggests that these individualist values have increased over the past few decades (Twenge & Foster, 2010). Ironically, the criteria by which individuals are viewed positively by "society" are often incompatible with the communal values that focus on benefitting other people and society as a whole. Of course, achievement and personal goal-striving have great value for individuals and society, so the problem is not that people value achievement and personal striving but rather that they consistently prioritize self-enhancement over self-transcendent values. And, the pervasive emphasis on achievement and personal success can contribute to egoism in the first place. Thus, to the extent that mindfulness promotes a hypo-egoic mindset that weakens the emphasis on self-enhancement, the more it promotes benevolent and universalist values (Baer, 2015; Hofmann, Grossman, & Hinton, 2011).

Reactions to undesired events

One widely documented effect of mindfulness is that it can transform and reduce people's reactions to undesired events (Arch & Craske, 2010; Creswell, Way, Eisenberger, & Lieberman, 2007; Erisman & Roemer, 2010; Weinstein, Brown, & Ryan, 2009). Indeed, many people first seek out mindfulness because of its reputation for reducing stress and negative emotions.

The effects of mindfulness on emotional balance and equanimity may arise from its impact on hypo-egoic mindsets. To the extent that strong emotional reactions are fed by abstract, symbolic, evaluative thoughts about oneself or one's past and future, the hypo-egoic nature of mindful thoughts (which are more present-focused, more concrete, less introspective, and less evaluative) leads people to react less strongly when things do not go the way they desire. Writers working from Buddhist perspectives often talk about mindfulness reducing people's "attachment" to particular outcomes (Ryan & Rigby, 2015; Sahdra, Shaver, & Brown, 2010). At its core, attachment can be viewed as an egoic insistence that life conform to one's wishes, an insistence that weakens when people's thoughts become hypo-egoic.

Mindfulness not only reduces the frequency of negative emotional reactions but also their intensity and duration. People often respond to events automatically before they consciously mull over what just happened. People who practice mindfulness often recognize these reactions before they become full-blown and adjust their thinking before being taken over by an emotion (Arch & Craske, 2010; Creswell, Way, Eisenberger, & Lieberman, 2007; see also Slutsky, Rahl, Lindsay, & Creswell, Chapter 6 in this volume). Again, hypo-egoic mindsets play a role in this process: Present-focused attention permits greater awareness of reactions as they unfold, and mindfulness training teaches skills that can be used to lower one's self-involvement. By telling themselves that their thoughts are not reality, psychologically distancing themselves from events, and engaging in other "cooling" operations (Lebois et al., 2015), people are in a better position to reappraise the situation and their initial response to it (Arch & Landy, 2015).

Mindfulness may reduce negative emotions via an additional hypo-egoic route: By reducing egoic reactions and fostering self-transcendent values, mindfulness helps people attain a broader perspective on events. When being hypo-egoic, people more easily recognize that everything isn't about them. As a result, their reactions are tempered by the realization that, in the big scheme of things, certain seemingly negative events are not only fairly trivial but also potentially desirable for other people. Various conceptualizations of wisdom make much the same point, suggesting that people who are less ego-involved in how events transpire have a broader, more discerning perspective that helps them make better decisions (Kross & Grossman, 2011; Pascual-Leone, 1990).

Although mindfulness reduces negatively valenced thoughts and attentional biases toward negative stimuli, its effects on positive thoughts are unclear. Traditional views suggest that mindfulness should reduce attentional and cognitive biases of all kinds and, thus, not function as a sort of cognitive reappraisal that puts a positive spin on negative events. However, some evidence suggests that mindfulness increases positive thoughts (Garland, Gaylord, & Fredrickson, 2011; Kiken & Shook, 2011), while some does not (Kiken & Shook, 2014). Given that it is often difficult to differentiate a "less negative" thought from a "more positive" one, the jury remains out on this issue.

Our view is that, when viewed as a hypo-egoic state, mindfulness should reduce both negative and positive biases in perception and judgement, but the affective impact of mindfulness should be most obvious with respect to negative emotions. The reason is straightforward: Although more present-focused and specific self-thoughts diminish the temporal and abstract thoughts that often create self-generated negative emotion, present-focused and specific thoughts are not, in and of themselves, more positive. Whatever increase in positive affect that people experience as a result of mindfulness appears generally due to lower negative self-thoughts and greater attention to events in the present moment rather than increased positive self-thoughts.

Defensiveness

A prevailing theme of both spiritual and psychological approaches is that mindfulness reduces defensive reactions to undesired social events such as criticism, disrespect, failure, and challenges to one's ideas, beliefs, and decisions (Brown, Ryan, & Creswell, 2007; Brown et al., 2008; Weinstein et al., 2009). Even when such events are trivial and have no tangible implications, people often react angrily, as if they are defending themselves against a major threat (Allen & Leary, 2010; Baumeister, Smart, & Boden, 1996; Leary, Diebels, Jongman-Sereno, & Fernandez, 2015).

But why does mindfulness reduce defensive reactions? The popular explanation is that these reactions occur when people's egos are threatened, so by reducing the person's ego, there is nothing to be threatened and, thus, nothing to defend. But the answer is probably more complicated than that, because the situations that provoke "defensive" reactions usually involve events that are not clearly threats to people's egos, as that term is usually defined. Rather, they involve situations in which people perceive that they are not treated as they believe they should be (Leary, Terry, Allen, & Tate, 2009). Although people have good reasons to insist that they are not harmed or disadvantaged by others, these reactions often stem from being personally invested in particular ideas about how one wants to be viewed and treated by others. The more that people think egoically about themselves and their goals, the more likely they are to be invested in outcomes and, thus, to take things personally when things do not transpire as they wish. Not only are mindful people less attached and egoic to begin with, but also when they do react defensively (old habits die hard), they are equipped to moderate their initial reaction with acceptance and equanimity.

Relationships to other people and the world

In addition to its effects on people's perceptions, self-views, and emotions, mindfulness promotes behaviours that facilitate interpersonal connections (Beitel, Ferrer, & Cecero, 2005; Brown et al., 2007). Again, hypo-egoicism plays a central role in these effects.

To understand why, consider that the egoic components of mindlessness – being excessively focused on one's own concerns, judging events in terms of personal outcomes, being entangled in one's thoughts and emotions, and being preoccupied with oneself and one's story – have negative effects on interactions and relationships with other people. People who are myopically focused on themselves are not as attuned to other people's perspectives and needs, and, thus, are less likely to be interested, empathic, or compassionate, whereas mindfulness is associated with greater attunement to others (Beitel, Ferrer, & Cecero, 2005; Birnie, Speca, & Carlson, 2010; Shapiro, Schwartz, & Bonner, 1998; Walsh & Shapiro, 2006). Indeed, egoicism can lead to overt selfishness, as manifested in an array of inconsiderate, irresponsible, and antisocial attitudes and behaviours that undermine relationships (Leary, Jongman-Sereno, Diebels, Hall, & Jones, 2015). Ironically, an egoic orientation can be detrimental not only to other people but also to oneself because highly egoic and unmindful people behave in ways that undermine the quality of their relationships – and they may even be devalued, avoided, or excluded for being disinterested, egocentric, or selfish.

In contrast, a hypo-egoic orientation promotes positive interactions and close relationships. People who are less self-preoccupied, egocentric, emotionally reactive, and defensive are regarded as more agreeable and enjoyable interactants. As a result, mindful people should be better interpersonal partners in both transient interactions and long-term relationships. Indeed, learning mindfulness reduces interpersonal problems (Gambrel & Keeling, 2010; Tloczynski & Tantriella, 1998), and people high in trait mindfulness show lower verbal aggression and negativity when discussing conflicts with their partner (Barnes et al., 2007; Gambrel & Keeling, 2010; Lakey, Kernis, Heppner, & Lance, 2008).

One important but understudied aspect of the appeal of mindful people involves the degree to which they are "present" when interacting with other people. With less inner self-talk, lower egoic preoccupation, and a focus on the present situation, mindful people have greater cognitive resources for attending to social interactions (Parker, Nelson, Epel, & Siegel, 2015). In addition, interacting mindfully should allow people to process social information more accurately and promote attunement to other people's intentions, reactions, and experiences (Parker et al., 2015). Interpersonal presence also promotes responsiveness, which is central to high-quality interactions and relationships (Reis & Clark, 2013) and likely leads other people to like, trust, and open up to mindful people (Carson, Carson, Gil, & Baucom, 2004). By enhancing presence and responsiveness, hypo-egoic mindsets make people more desirable social interactants and relationship partners (Karremans, Schellekens, & Kappen, 2015; Karremans & Kappen, Chapter 8 in this volume).

As noted, hypo-egoicism is associated with self-construals that include one's connections with other people and the natural world (Maslow, 1971; Wayment et al., 2014). In perceiving their connections with others, mindful people are likely to resonate with and connect to a wider array of other people. Having a broad, all-inclusive identity that incorporates both close and distant others is associated with greater kindness, forgiveness, compassion, and placing greater value on social relationships (Leary et al., 2008). Including others in one's identity has also been associated with empathy, perspective taking, and prosocial behaviour (Cialdini, Brown, Lewis, Luce, & Neuberg, 1997).

Meta-cognitive mediators of mindfulness effects

Although these effects of mindfulness appear to be mediated by the direct effects of hypo-egoic mindsets on perception, self-relevant thought, and emotion, some effects may result not from hypo-egoicism (or mindfulness) per se but rather from exposure to the philosophical, spiritual, or psychological frameworks in which mindfulness training is usually embedded.

Historically, people learned mindfulness and other meditation practices in the context of Eastern philosophical, spiritual, or religious traditions involving Buddhism, Taoism, Hinduism, or one of their offshoots. These traditions are characterized by a set of assumptions regarding the nature of reality, human suffering, the self, well-being, and morality. As a result, people who learn mindfulness within these traditions invariably acquire not only a new set of cognitive/attentional skills but also new beliefs about themselves and the world, many of which rely on hypo-egoic ideas. Given this, the practice of mindfulness is typically associated with a certain worldview, which makes it difficult to determine the degree to which effects of "practicing mindfulness" are due to mindfulness per se versus the adoption of new beliefs.

As it has been secularized in the West, mindfulness is often taught largely outside the context of the philosophical, spiritual, or religious frameworks in which it has historically been embedded. Even so, secular mindfulness training is nonetheless accompanied by a psychological worldview, rooted partly in its Eastern origins, that provides a context for novice practitioners to understand themselves, the source of their problems, and the processes by which mindfulness is supposed to reduce those difficulties.

Thus, mindfulness is always taught within a framework that provides novel information and insights; indeed, it's hard to imagine an instructor teaching mindfulness without saying anything whatsoever about what it is, what it is supposed to do, or how it works. Whether framed in spiritual/religious or psychological terms, these beliefs and the insights they stimulate probably contribute to some of the effects that are typically attributed to the practice or trait of mindfulness itself. For example, as instructors teach students tactics for being in the present, they typically describe the detrimental effects of paying excessive attention to past and future. As a result, we do not know how much of the effects of mindfulness are due to the practice of a mindful state as opposed to knowledge about it and the resulting shift in views of oneself and the world.

We are unaware of research that has directly examined these two distinct influences separately, but existing data present a muddy picture. Using a sample of participants with major depressive disorder, Williams et al. (2014) compared the effects of standard Mindfulness-Based Cognitive Therapy (MBCT) to a cognitive psychological education (CPE) program that included all aspects of the MBCT program except the direct cultivation of mindfulness through exercises and meditation. Results showed that full-blown MBCT was no more effective than CPE, suggesting that the meditative component did not enhance treatment effectiveness. However, unlike the findings of similar studies, MBCT was no more effective than treatment-as-usual, which raises questions about its efficacy in this instance. Yet Crane et al. (2014) found that the amount of time that participants in a MBCT program practiced meditation at home was strongly associated with lower relapse, suggesting that the meditative component was important.

Although research is clearly needed to explore the impact of various aspects of mindfulness training, from a practical standpoint, it may not matter. A mindfulness intervention may be notably beneficial without us having any idea regarding how much of its effect is due to learning how to engage a particular mental state as opposed to learning new ways to think about one's mind or one's relationship to the world.

Yet, from a scientific standpoint, it makes a considerable difference if we want to understand why mindfulness does what it does. One can imagine an experiment with three different "mindfulness" interventions: one that teaches the conceptual foundations of mindfulness but with no instruction in the practice of mindfulness itself, one that teaches mindfulness practice but with no conceptual framing whatsoever, and one that includes both information and practice (as mindfulness is actually taught). Such a study could show the relative effects of the pedagogical versus experiential elements of mindfulness training on various outcomes of mindfulness.

Conclusions

The psychological and interpersonal effects of mindfulness can be understood most generally in terms of a change in self-focus and self-preoccupation that can be characterized as hypo-egoic. In promoting a state in which self-relevant thoughts are fewer, more present-focused, more concrete, less introspective, and less evaluative than usual, mindfulness minimizes the kinds of self-thoughts that elicit and maintain undesired emotion, changes people's views of themselves and their relations to others, reduces defensiveness, fosters interpersonal presence, and strengthens social connections. Of course, these are just some of the more pronounced effects of trait and state mindfulness, and additional work is needed to explore more fully the role of hypo-egoic mindsets in the cognitive, emotional, and behavioural features of mindfulness.

References

Allen, A. B., & Leary, M. R. (2010). Reactions to others' selfish actions in the absence of tangible consequences. *Basic and Applied Social Psychology, 32*, 26–34.

Arch, J. J., & Craske, M. G. (2010). Laboratory stressors in clinically anxious and non-anxious individuals: The moderating role of mindfulness. *Behaviour Research and Therapy, 48*, 495–505.

Arch, J. J., & Landy, L. N. (2015). Emotional benefits of mindfulness. In K. W. Brown, J. D. Creswell, & R. M. Ryan (Eds.), *Handbook of mindfulness: Theory, research, and practice* (pp. 208–224). New York: Guilford Press.

Baer, R. (2015). Ethics, values, virtues, and character strengths in mindfulness-based interventions: A psychological science perspective. *Mindfulness, 6*, 956–969.

Barnes, S., Brown, K. W., Krusemark, E., Campbell, W. K., & Rogge, R. D. (2007). The role of mindfulness in romantic relationship satisfaction and responses to relationship stress. *Journal of Marriage and Family Therapy, 33*, 482–500.

Baumeister, R. F. (1991). *Escaping the self: Alcoholism, spirituality, masochism, and other flights from the burden of selfhood.* New York: Basic Books.

Baumeister, R. F., Smart, L., & Boden, J. M. (1996). Relation of threatened egotism to violence and aggression: The dark side of high self-esteem. *Psychological Review, 103*, 5–33.

Beitel, M., Ferrer, E., & Cecero, J. J. (2005). Psychological mindedness and awareness of self and others. *Journal of Clinical Psychology, 61*, 739–750.

Birnie, K., Speca, M., & Carlson, L. E. (2010). Exploring self-compassion and empathy in the context of Mindfulness-Based Stress Reduction (MBSR). *Stress and Health: Journal of the International Society for the Investigation of Stress, 26*, 359–371.

Bishop, S. R., Lau, M., Shapiro, S., Carlson, L., Anderson, N. D., Carmody, J., . . . Devins, G. (2004). Mindfulness: A proposed operational definition. *Clinical Psychology: Science, and Practice, 11*, 230–241.

Boisselier, J. (1993). *The wisdom of the Buddha.* New York: Abrams.

Brewer, J. A., Elwafi, H. M., & Davis, J. H. (2013). Craving to quit: Psychological models and neurobiological mechanisms of mindfulness training as treatment for addiction. *Psychology of Addictive Behaviors, 27*, 366–379.

Brown, K. W., Creswell, J. D., & Ryan, R. M. (Eds.) (2015). *Handbook of mindfulness: Theory, research, and practice.* New York, NY: Guilford.

Brown, K. W., & Leary, M. R. (2016). The emergence of scholarship and science on hypo-egoic phenomena. In K. W. Brown & M. R. Leary (Eds.), *The Oxford handbook of hypo-egoic phenomena* (pp. 3–16). New York: Oxford University Press.

Brown, K. W., Ryan, R. M., & Creswell, J. D. (2007). Mindfulness: Theoretical foundations and evidence for its salutary effects. *Psychological Inquiry, 18*, 211–237.

Brown, K. W., Ryan, R. M., Creswell, J. D., & Niemiec, C. P. (2008). Beyond me: Mindful responses to social threat. In H. A. Wayment & J. J. Bauer (Eds.), *Transcending self- interest: Psychological explorations of the quiet ego* (pp. 75–84). Washington, DC: American Psychological Association.

Carlson, E. N. (2013). Overcoming the barriers to self-knowledge: Mindfulness as a path to seeing yourself as you really are. *Perspectives in Psychological Science, 8*, 173–186.

Carson, J. W., Carson, K. M., Gil, K., & Baucom, D. H. (2004). Mindfulness-based relationship enhancement. *Behavior Therapy, 35*, 471–494.

Cialdini, R. B., Brown, S. L., Lewis, B. P., Luce, C., & Neuberg, S. L. (1997). Reinterpreting the empathy-altruism relationship: When one into one equals oneness. *Journal of Personality and Social Psychology, 52*, 749–758.

Crane, C., Crane, R. S., Eames, C., Fennell, M. J., Silverton, S., Williams, J. M. G., & Barnhofer, T. (2014). The effects of amount of home meditation practice in mindfulness based cognitive therapy on hazard of relapse to depression in the staying well after depression trial. *Behaviour Research and Therapy, 63*, 17–24.

Creswell, J. D., Way, B. M., Eisenberger, N. I., & Lieberman, M. D. (2007). Neural correlates of dispositional mindfulness during affect labeling. *Psychosomatic Medicine, 69*, 560–565.

Duval, T. S., & Wicklund, R. A. (1972). *A theory of objective self-awareness.* New York: Academic.

Emanuel, A. S., Updegraff, J. A., Kalmbach, D. A., & Ciesla, J. A. (2010). The role of mindfulness facets in affective forecasting. *Personality and Individual Differences, 49*, 815–818.

Epstein, M. (1995). *Thoughts without a thinker: Psychotherapy from a Buddhist perspective.* New York, NY: Basic Books.

Erisman, S. M., & Roemer, L. (2010). A preliminary investigation of the effects of experimentally induced mindfulness on emotional responding to film clips. *Emotion, 10*, 72–82.

Farb, N. A. S., Segal, Z. V., Mayberg, H., Bean, J., McKeon, D., Fatima, Z., & Anderson, A. K. (2007). Attending to the present: Mindfulness meditation reveals distinct neural modes of self-reference. *Social Cognitive and Affective Neuroscience, 2*, 313–322.

Galin, D. (2003). The concepts "self," "person," and "I" in Western psychology and Buddhism. In B. A. Wallace (Ed.), *Buddhism and science: Breaking new ground* (pp. 107–142). New York: Columbia University Press.

Gambrel, L. E., & Keeling, M. L. (2010). Relational aspects of mindfulness: Implications for the practice of marriage and family therapy. *Contemporary Family Therapy, 32*, 412–426.

Garland, E., Gaylord, S., & Fredrickson, B. L. (2011). Positive reappraisal mediates the stress-reductive effects of mindfulness: An upward spiral process. *Mindfulness, 2*, 59–67.

Hargus, E., Crane, C., Barnhofer, T., & Williams, J. M. G. (2010). Effects of mindfulness on meta-awareness and specificity of describing prodromal symptoms in suicidal depression. *Emotion, 10*, 34–42.

Hill, C. L. M., & Updegraff, J. A. (2012). Mindfulness and its relationship to emotional regulation. *Emotion, 12*, 81–90.

Hofmann, S. G., Grossman, P., Hinton, D. E. (2011). Loving-kindness and compassion meditation: Potential for psychological interventions. *Clinical Psychology Review, 31*, 1126–1132.

Hölzel, B. K., Lazar, S. W., Gard, T., Schuman-Olivier, Z., Vago, D. R., & Ott, U. (2011). How does mindfulness meditation work? Proposing mechanisms of action from a conceptual and neural perspective. *Perspectives on Psychological Science, 6*, 537–559.

Kabat-Zinn, J. (1994). *Wherever you go, there you are.* New York: Hyperion.

Karremans, J. C., Schellekens, M. P. J., & Kappen, G. (2015). Bridging the sciences on mindfulness and relationships: A research agenda. *Personality and Social Psychology Review, 21,* 29–49.

Kiken, L. G., Garland, E. L., Bluth, K., Paisson, O. S., & Gaylord, S. A. (2015). From a state to a trait: Trajectories of state mindfulness in meditation during intervention predict changes in trait mindfulness. *Personality and Individual Differences, 81,* 41–46.

Kiken, L. G., & Shook, N. J. (2011). Looking up: Mindfulness increases positive judgments and reduces negativity bias. *Social Psychological and Personality Science, 2,* 425–431.

Kiken, L. G., & Shook, N. J. (2014). Does mindfulness attenuate thoughts emphasizing negativity but not positivity? *Journal of Research in Personality, 53,* 22–30.

Kross, E., & Grossmann, I. (2011). Boosting wisdom: Distance from the self enhances wise reasoning, attitudes, and behavior. *Journal of Experimental Psychology: General, 141,* 43–48.

Lakey, C. E., Kernis, M. H., Heppner, W. L., & Lance, C. E. (2008). Individual differences in authenticity and mindfulness as predictors of verbal defensiveness. *Journal of Research in Personality, 42,* 230–238.

Leary, M. R. (2004). Digging deeper: The fundamental nature of "self-conscious" emotions. *Psychological Inquiry, 15*(2), 129–131.

Leary, M. R., & Buttermore, N. E. (2003). Evolution of the human self: Tracing the natural history of self-awareness. *Journal for the Theory of Social Behaviour, 33,* 365–404.

Leary, M. R., & Diebels, K. (2013). Hypo-egoic states: Features and developmental processes. In D. M. McInerney, H. W. Marsh, R. G. Craven, & F. Guay (Eds.), *Theory driving research: New wave perspectives on self-processes and human development* (pp. 31–52). Charlotte, NC: Information Age Publishing.

Leary, M. R., Diebels, K. J., Jongman-Sereno, K. P., & Fernandez, X. D. (2015). Why seemingly trivial events sometimes evoke strong emotional reactions: The role of social exchange rule violations. *Journal of Social Psychology, 155,* 559–575.

Leary, M. R., Estrada, M. J., & Allen, A. B. (2009). The analogue-I and the analogue-Me: The avatars of the self. *Self and Identity, 8,* 147–161.

Leary, M. R., Jongman-Sereno, K. P., Diebels, K. J., Hall, A. N., & Jones, C. E. (2015). *Selfishness predicts a broad range of inconsiderate, manipulative, unethical, and antisocial attitudes and behaviors.* Unpublished manuscript, Duke University.

Leary, M. R., & Terry, M. L. (2012). Hypo-egoic mindsets: Antecedents and implications of quieting the self. In M. R. Leary & J. P. Tangney (Eds.), *Handbook of self and identity* (2nd ed.; pp. 268–288). New York: Guilford.

Leary, M. R., Terry, M. L., Allen, A. B., & Tate, E. B. (2009). The concept of ego threat in social and personality psychology: In ego threat a viable scientific construct? *Personality and Social Psychology Review, 13,* 151–164.

Leary, M. R., Tipsord, J., & Tate, E. B. (2008). Allo-inclusive identity: Incorporating the natural and social worlds into one's sense of self. In H. Wayment & J. Bauer (Eds.), *Transcending self-interest: Psychological explorations of the quiet ego* (pp. 137–148). Washington, DC: American Psychological Association.

Lebois, L. A. M., Papies, E. K., Gopinath, K., Cabanban, R., Quigley, K. S., Krishnamurthy, V., . . . Barsalou, L. W. (2015). A shift in perspective: Decentering through mindful attention to imagined stressful events. *Neuropsychologia, 75,* 505–524.

Martin, L. (1999). I-D compensation theory: Some implications of trying to satisfy immediate-return needs in a delayed-return culture. *Psychological Inquiry, 10,* 195–208.

Maslow, A. (1971). *The farther reaches of human nature.* New York: The Viking Press.

Mulcahy, N. J., & Call, J. (2006). Apes save tools for future use. *Science, 312,* 1038–1040.

Papies, E. K., Pronk, T. M., Keesman, M., & Barsalou, L. W. (2015). The benefits of simply observing: Mindful attention modulates the link between motivation and behavior. *Journal of Personality and Social Psychology, 108*, 148.

Parker, S. C., Nelson, B. W., Epel, E. S., & Siegel, D. J. (2015). The science of presence: A central mediator of the interpersonal benefits of mindfulness. In K. W. Brown, J. D. Creswell, & R. M. Ryan (Eds.), *Handbook of mindfulness: Theory, research, and practice* (pp. 225–244). New York: Guilford Press.

Pascual-Leone, J. (1990). An essay on wisdom: Toward organism process that make it possible. In R. J. Sternberg (Ed.), *Wisdom, its nature, origins, and development* (pp. 244–278). Cambridge, UK: Cambridge University Press.

Phelan, J. P. (2010). Mindfulness as presence. *Mindfulness, 1*, 131–134.

Reis, H. T., & Clark, M. S. (2013). Responsiveness. In J. A. Simpson & L. Campbell (Eds.), *The Oxford handbook of close relationships* (pp. 400–423). New York: Oxford University Press.

Ryan, R. M., & Rigby, C. S. (2015). Did the Buddha have a self? No-self, self, and mindfulness in Buddhist thought and Western psychologies. In K. W. Brown, J. D. Creswell, & R. M. Ryan (Eds.), *Handbook of mindfulness: Theory, research, and practice* (pp. 245–265). New York: Guilford Press.

Sahdra, B. K., Shaver, P. R., & Brown, K. W. (2010). A scale to measure nonattachment: A Buddhist complement to Western research on attachment and adaptive functioning. *Journal of Personality Assessment, 92*, 116–127.

Schwartz, S. H. (1994). Are there universal aspects in the content and structure of values? *Journal of Social Issues, 50*, 19–45.

Shapiro, S. L., Schwartz, G. E., & Bonner, G. (1998). Effects of mindfulness-based stress reduction on medical and premedical students. *Journal of Behavioral Medicine, 21*, 581–599.

Tloczynski, J., & Tantriella, M. (1998). A comparison of the effects of Zen breath meditation or relaxation on college adjustment. *Psychologia: An International Journal of Psychology in the Orient, 41*, 32–43.

Twenge, J. M., & Foster, J. D. (2010). Birth cohort increases in narcissistic personality traits among American college students, 1982–2009. *Social Psychological and Personality Science, 1*, 99–106.

Walsh, R., & Shapiro, S. L. (2006). The meeting of meditative disciplines and Western psychology: A mutually enriching dialogue. *American Psychologist, 61*, 227–239.

Watkins, E. R. (2015). Mindfulness in the context of processing mode theory. In K. W. Brown, J. D. Creswell, & R. M. Ryan (Eds.), *Handbook of mindfulness: Theory, research, and practice* (pp. 90–111). New York: Guilford Press.

Wayment, H. A., Bauer, J. J., & Sylaska, K. (2014). The Quiet Ego Scale: Measuring the compassionate self-identity. *Journal of Happiness Studies, 16*, 999–1033.

Weinstein, N., Brown, K. W., & Ryan, R. M. (2009). A multi-method examination of the effects of mindfulness on stress attribution, coping, and emotional well-being. *Journal of Research in Personality, 43*, 374–385.

Williams, J. M. G., Crane, C., Barnhofer, T., Brennan, K., Duggan, D. S., Fennell, M. J., . . . Russell, I. T. (2014). Mindfulness-based cognitive therapy for preventing relapse in recurrent depression: A randomized dismantling trial. *Journal of Consulting and Clinical Psychology, 82*, 275–286.

5

HOW MINDFULNESS ENHANCES SELF-CONTROL

Nathaniel Elkins-Brown, Rimma Teper, and Michael Inzlicht

Self-control features prominently in the everyday life of the modern human. Eating healthy, exercising consistently, completing chores, doing our jobs well, and remaining patient in trying circumstances are just a few examples of behaviours that self-control makes possible. A growing body of research suggests that mindfulness training and mindful personality traits are related to better self-control, both in and outside of the laboratory (see Karremans & Kappen, Chapter 8 in this volume; Mrazek et al., Chapter 10 in this volume; Papies, Chapter 7 in this volume). Here, we elaborate on the mechanics behind this relationship.

Converging evidence suggests that the present-moment awareness and non-judgemental acceptance intrinsic to mindfulness enhances one's sensitivity to the affective cues that direct self-control processes. Rapid and transient affect is produced when one is at risk of not meeting one's goals, and this affect serves as a signal that alerts the brain that the self-control is needed. As the cultivation of mindfulness promotes the employment of a non-judgemental attention towards primary affective and sensory experiences (e.g. Farb, Segal, & Anderson, 2013), mindfulness training enhances affect's ability to energize controlled processes in the service of goal-directed behaviour. In the following chapter, we discuss new findings that illuminate how affect guides self-control processes, and how the cultivation of mindfulness refines the relationship between affect and self-control.

Self-control and mindfulness training

We define self-control – referred to more colloquially as willpower and more formally as cognitive control – as the mental processes that allow one to override thoughts, emotions, or behaviours that differ with one's overarching goals. At its core, self-control is instigated when individuals experience conflicts between opposing desires, competing response tendencies, or anticipated and actual outcomes. Controlled processes may be initiated, for example, when someone on a diet is offered a delicious but unhealthy piece of cake; or when a quitting smoker is handed a cigarette at a party; or even when a psychology study participant is tempted to *read* a colour word in a Stroop task, rather than correctly name the font colour. These situations consist of immediate desires or prepotent responses (e.g. eating the cake, smoking the cigarette, reading the word) that conflict with behaviours that are consistent with overarching goals (e.g. "eat healthy", "don't smoke", "name the font colour"). Effective self-control can be thought of as the successful inhibition and substitution of these automatic behaviours with more deliberate behaviours that are in line with one's long-standing goals (see also Barsalou, Chapter 3 in this volume).

This definition of self-control can be most closely related to the inhibitory component or aspect of what researchers call the *executive functions*. These executive functions are comprised of the "higher-level" cognitive mechanisms that the brain uses to control other "lower-level" processes, largely in the service of complex behaviour like planning, reasoning, problem-solving, and goal pursuit. In one prominent model, the primary executive functions include maintaining information in working memory, flexibly switching between task sets or rules, and – most germane to our definition of self-control – inhibiting or suppressing dominant responses (Miyake et al., 2000; Miyake & Friedman, 2012). Our discussion of self-control in this chapter will be most closely related to this third executive function: the inhibition of prepotent responses and desires. This definition allows us to distinguish it from similar constructs like self-regulation (Vohs & Baumeister, 2011), which more broadly refers to any regulatory behaviour motivated by abstract and self-related goals. Through the inhibition of prepotent and impulsive behaviour, however, we can classify self-control as being one of a number of ways that self-regulation may be accomplished (Fujita, 2011).

Importantly, mindfulness training has been associated with enhanced executive functioning. In the laboratory, for example, meditators show less interference from conflict and make fewer errors in the Stroop task than controls (Chan & Woollacott, 2007; Moore & Malinowski, 2009; Teper & Inzlicht, 2013; Van den Hurk et al., 2010; Wenk-Sormaz, 2005). Similar improvements have also been observed in the Attention Network Test (Fan et al., 2002), where meditators show an enhanced capacity for monitoring conflict (Jha, Krompinger, & Baim, 2007; Tang et al., 2007). In both of these tasks, individuals must override learned, natural response tendencies that conflict with their intentions. This kind of conflict parallels the self-control struggles that people face outside of the laboratory, where desires and cravings conflict with long-term goals. Accordingly, more hours of formal and informal meditative practice have been related to better outcomes in smoking cessation (e.g. Elwafi et al., 2013; Tang, Tang, & Posner, 2013) and alcohol use (e.g. Bowen et al., 2006), and preliminary evidence suggests that mindfulness meditation may be an effective treatment for substance abuse disorders (Chiesa & Serretti, 2014).

So, how then does mindfulness meditation bring about its fortuitous effects on self-control? The overarching goal of mindfulness is to attend to moment-to-moment experiences with a non-judgemental and non-elaborative mindset. We propose that in cultivating greater attention and acceptance towards thoughts and feelings in the experiential field, mindfulness meditators are better prepared to acknowledge moment-to-moment affect that signals the need for self-control (Teper & Inzlicht, 2013). To explore this idea further, we must first understand the emotional underpinnings of self-control processes.

Emotion and emotional episodes

Historically, emotions have been cast as a principal antagonist of self-control and of cognition more broadly. From Stoic philosophy, to Cartesian dualism, to the Freudian psyche, and into modern theory (e.g. Metcalfe & Mischel, 1999), emotions have been variously described as opposing rationality, deliberation, contemplation, calculation, and virtuous decision-making. However, most contemporary theorists do not view cognition and emotion as opposable or mutually exclusive constructs at all. Indeed, many have suggested that they are fully integrated and only minimally decomposable (e.g. Frijda, 1988; Ochsner & Gross, 2005; Parrott & Schulkin, 1993; Pessoa, 2008). Naturally, while research in the past two decades has extensively outlined the cognitive and neural underpinnings of self-control (e.g. Botvinick, Braver, Barch, Carter, & Cohen, 2001; Carver & Scheier, 1998; Hofmann, Friese, & Strack, 2009), recent work has also characterized self-control as an emotional process that may be likened to an emotional episode (Inzlicht, Bartholow, & Hirsh, 2015; Saunders, Milyavskaya, & Inzlicht, 2015).

We can define an emotional episode as consisting of an antecedent event of some motivational significance – such as the appearance of a bear while hiking, or being kissed by a intimate partner – that produces a cascade of physiological, phenomenological, behavioural, and cognitive changes apropos of that antecedent event (Russell & Barrett, 1999). We are likely to undergo a complex series of changes across our physical and experiential systems upon, for example, smelling something rancid when opening the refrigerator after a vacation. Physiologically, we may observe variations in heart rate, skin conductance, and respiration (Stark, Walter, Schienle, & Vaitl, 2005); phenomenally, we may experience revulsion and a strong desire to avoid the smell; behaviourally, we may physically recoil and express disgust in our bodies and faces (Stark et al., 2005; Vrana, 1993); and cognitively, we may engage in processes like attribution and appraisal to determine the source to the smell ("the potato salad") and what to do next ("throw it out!"; Schachter & Singer, 1962; Gross, 1998; Russell, 2003). In this way, we can view emotional episodes as states that prepare individuals to act or respond to motivationally significant stimuli in the immediate environment, and facilitate goal-related action concerning those stimuli (Frijda, 1988).

In what way may one consider self-control an emotional process? We propose that *conflict* between goals and desires can be considered the antecedent event of an emotional episode, where rapid and transient negative affect is produced as a function of the context and magnitude of that conflict (Inzlicht, Bartholow, & Hirsh,

2015). This conflict-related negative affect serves to mobilize self-control processes by orienting individuals toward the source of the affect (i.e. the conflict), alerting them to the possibility that their goals are at risk of not being met, and motivating them to engage in behaviour that will reduce the negative affect. Thus, just as emotions arise as an adaptive response to motivationally significant events in general, this rapid and transient negative affect arises as an adaptive response to conflicts.

Control begins with conflict, and conflict produces negative affect

Evidence across multiple domains of scientific inquiry suggests that conflict-related negative affect is instrumental to self-control (Inzlicht et al., 2015). From social psychology to cognitive neuroscience, a diverse literature supports the idea that negative affect from conflict acts as a kind of signal or "alarm" that current behaviour is no longer sufficient for maintaining goal pursuit, and that changes and adjustments are necessary for goals to be met. Accordingly, the kinds of conflicts that can produce this negative affect are broad, and go beyond abstract goal conflicts: They can include conflicts between opposing impulses, between competing response tendencies, between incompatible mental representations, between expected and actual outcomes, and so forth. In all cases, conflicts that fail to produce enough of this negative affect reduce the chance that one will shift behaviour from routine and automatic to deliberate and controlled.

We can see this idea reflected in behavioural and pharmacological work done in humans and rodents, for example, where *revised reinforcement sensitivity theory* has described an instrumental role for negative affect in control. In this theory, conflicts between goals of the appetitive and avoidance motivational systems produce anxiety, which inhibits present behaviour and initiates a process of risk assessment to determine subsequent behaviour (Gray & McNaughton, 2000). If a smoker is trying to quit and is offered a cigarette, for example, their overarching avoidance-goal to quit smoking will conflict with their automatic approach-goal to smoke. This conflict produces anxiety, which facilitates the inhibition of prepotent behaviour (smoking cigarettes, in this case) as the brain assesses whether "smoking" or "not-smoking" is the most optimal course of action. In support of this theory, researchers have shown that septo-hippocampal lesions and anti-anxiety drugs – but not anti-fear ones – impair inhibition and conflict resolution in response to goal conflicts (Perkins et al., 2009; Perkins et al., 2013). In revised reinforcement sensitivity theory, conflict-related anxiety acts as both an inhibitor of current behaviour and an initiator of risk assessment, providing clear support for the notion that negative affect can be instrumental in self-control processes.

Research in cognitive neuroscience also points toward an integral role for anxiety and negative affect in self-control, where errors in task performance constitute their own kind of conflict. The consumption of alcohol, for example – which has potent anxiolytic properties (e.g. Donohue, Curtin, Patrick, & Lang, 2007; Levenson, Sher, Grossman, Newman, & Newlin, 1980; see also Lee,

Greely, & Oei, 1999) – has been shown to impair behavioural and neural measures of error-monitoring during self-control tasks (Bailey, Bartholow, Saults, & Lust, 2014; Bartholow, Henry, Lust, Saults, & Wood, 2012). In these studies, participants performed a self-control task following the administration of an alcoholic, placebo, or non-alcoholic beverage. They also provided reports of their emotional state and perceived accuracy in terms of task performance. The authors found that both subjective and physiological measures of negative emotion mediated the relationship between beverage consumption and behavioural adjustments after errors, such that consumers of alcohol reported less negative emotion and less post-error adjustment compared to consumers of other beverages. Critically, alcohol consumers were just as accurate at realizing when they had made errors as the other beverage consumer groups, suggesting that their reduced adjustments after errors could not be explained by impairments in attention or awareness (Easdon, Izenberg, Armilio, Yu, & Alain, 2005; Ridderinkhof et al., 2002; Yeung, Ralph, & Nieuwenhuis, 2007). It appeared that the negative emotions that arose from making a self-control error – and not simply the awareness of having made one – were important for being able to compensate after failures of self-control.

Reinforcement sensitivity theory and the effects of alcohol on error-monitoring comprise only a fraction of the literature that supports an instrumental role for negative affect in self-control. However, each of these areas of investigation illustrate a unique mechanism by which negative affect can facilitate controlled processing. In the case of reinforcement sensitivity theory, negative affect disrupts automatic or routine behaviour and draws attention toward goal conflicts. In the case of error-monitoring, the aversive quality of negative affect motivates individuals to adjust their behaviour. These unique mechanisms will be important to remember in the next sections of this chapter, where we will explore how two major facets of mindfulness – moment-to-moment awareness and non-judgemental acceptance – enhance self-control through conflict-related negative affect.

Awareness and acceptance of conflict-related affect

A central feature of mindfulness is a present-moment awareness of elements in the experiential field (Brown & Ryan, 2003; Cardaciotto, Herbert, Forman, Moitra, & Farrow, 2008; Deikman, 1996; Roemer & Orsillo, 2003). During mindfulness meditation, practitioners actively deploy their attention towards primary visceral sensations, emerging thoughts, and affective feeling-states of the present moment. Whether focusing attention on the breath in many traditional forms of meditation (e.g. Hart, 2011), or focusing on ruminating thoughts in mindfulness-based therapy, or focusing on the whole viscera in the "body scans" of secular practice, mindfulness includes a directed, inquisitive, and open attention to interoceptive signals and internal experiences.

Importantly, this attention is also accompanied by a fundamental attitude of non-judgement, non-elaboration, and acceptance (Hayes, 1994; Kabat-Zinn, 1994; Marlatt & Kristeller, 1999; Roemer & Orsillo, 2003). When spontaneous thoughts, emotions, or memories inevitably draw attention away from the present moment, practitioners are instructed to be open, equanimous, and non-reactive towards these experiences, allowing them to capture attention without extended elaboration, narrativization, or regulation. In effect, mindfulness cultivates an awareness and acceptance to momentary experiences without letting any one sequence of sensations, emotions, memories, or thoughts dominate the experiential field.

How do these two elements of mindfulness – *awareness* and *acceptance* – support the implementation of control? First, through repeatedly centring attention on internal sensations during meditation, individuals develop the capacity to become spontaneously aware of those sensations also outside of meditation, in their everyday lives and happenings. When this cultivated awareness draws conscious attention to the negative affect of goal conflicts, individuals have greater leverage in responding to that affect in a controlled manner (Barrett, Gross, Christensen, & Benvenuto, 2001). Second, through repeatedly considering moment-to-moment sensations with a mindset of curiosity and acceptance, physical and experiential magnitude increases, which affords a greater chance of evolving towards whatever functional ends that are adaptively served. In the case of self-control, a cultivated acceptance elevates negative affect's propensity to disrupt routine behaviour, draw attention to goal conflicts, and motivate behavioural adjustments. When awareness and acceptance are then combined, the individual's chance of detecting transient affect and responding to it in a goal-congruent manner becomes greatly improved.

Awareness

Many mindfulness practices involve a sustained attention to subtle interoceptive sensations, such as respiration, proprioception, affective "twinges", and so forth. If it is the case that mindfulness cultivates a superior awareness of internal sensations, then we might expect to see this refinement reflected in the brains, behaviour, and subjective experiences of those who cultivate it. Accordingly, a number of studies have described such an enhanced sensitivity among mindfulness practitioners, suggesting that they may also have a greater chance of detecting and identifying the negative affect intrinsic to goal conflicts.

For example, when their self-reports of tactile sensation during meditation are compared to objective measures of tactile sensitivity, expert meditators display better introspective accuracy compared to novices (Fox et al., 2012). Meditators may also perform better on interoceptive breathing tasks than controls (Daubenmier, Sze, Kerr, Kemeny, & Mehling, 2013; Levinson, Stoll, Kindy, Merry, & Davidson, 2014), although this work requires further validation (Davidson & Kaszniak, 2015). In a task where participants reported their emotional reactions to masked and unmasked pictures, long-term meditators with greater "emotional clarity" were more likely to accurately discriminate the valence of masked, unpleasant stimuli (Nielsen & Kaszniak, 2006) than non-meditators, or meditators with less emotional clarity.

These subjective and behavioural differences are also supported by neuroimaging studies. When asked to focus on the breath or bodily experiences, individuals with mindfulness training have increased activation in neural regions associated with primary viscerosomatic sensation, like the insula, inferior parietal lobule, and somatosensory cortex (Farb et al., 2007; Farb et al., 2013). Similarly, when subjected to unpleasant electrical shocks, meditators show greater activation in regions related to the primary processing of pain, like the anterior cingulate cortex, thalamus, and insula (Gard et al., 2012; Grant, Courtemanche, & Rainville, 2011). In all of these studies, this increased activity was concurrent with decreases in areas related to rumination, evaluation, and self-referential processes, such as the medial prefrontal cortex, amygdala, and hippocampus. This suggests that mindfulness specifically fosters an interoceptive awareness of sensation that is not obfuscated by cognitive appraisals (Farb et al., 2015) or by high-order regulatory processes. Thus, we suspect that meditators and mindful individuals are uniquely predisposed to become aware of the sensory and affective cues that signal the need for self-control, in spite of the simultaneous presence of other sensations and thoughts in the experiential field.

Once individuals become aware of conflict-related affect, they may have a better chance of responding to it in a goal-congruent manner. Mindfulness is correlated with greater emotional awareness (Baer, Smith, & Allen, 2004) and differentiation (Hill & Updegraff, 2012), both of which are related to positive regulatory outcomes (e.g. Erbas, Ceulemans, Lee Pe, Koval, & Kuppens, 2014). When individuals become aware of emotions and can distinguish between them ("I feel *angry*"), they facilitate their adaptive regulation ("I need to *calm down*"; Barrett et al., 2001; see also Karremans & Kappen, Chapter 8 in this volume).

However, awareness of negative emotions does not always lead to adaptive outcomes. Panic disorder is associated with heightened interoceptive awareness (Ehlers & Breuer, 1992, 1996), for example, and attention to pain is related to emotional distress and psychosocial disability in patients with chronic pain (McCracken, 1997). It may be the case that interoceptive awareness can just as easily promote rumination and anxiety as it does goal-congruent regulation. Thus, we argue that awareness is best accompanied by another fundamental component of mindfulness in order to facilitate self-control: non-judgemental acceptance.

Acceptance

While enhanced awareness may bring negative affect into the forefront of consciousness and allow people to respond to it adaptively, a keen negative affect can mobilize control without conscious awareness. We propose that a non-reactive acceptance toward conflict-related negative affect can amplify its instrumental quality, in that "accepted" affect has an intensity and clarity that is more likely to disrupt routine behaviour, draw attention to conflict, and motivate compensatory control than affect that is not explicitly accepted. Whether through the attenuation of cognitive processes that might diminish it, or simply through increasing sensitivity to negative affect, acceptance nurtures the functional capacity of negative affect to recruit self-control.

This facilitative effect of acceptance is perhaps best illustrated in studies of error-monitoring, where participants' errors in self-control tasks are accompanied by an evoked brain potential called the *error-related negativity* (ERN; Gehring, Goss, Coles, Meyer, & Donchin, 1993). The ERN is thought to represent the activation of a neuroaffective system that monitors and adjusts for conflicts and errors, and its magnitude reflects both cognitive (Botvinick et al., 2001; Holroyd & Coles, 2002) and affective (Hajcak & Foti, 2008) features of making an error. Some theorists argue, for example, that the ERN at least partially represents a distress- or threat-related response to errors (Weinberg, Riesel, & Hajcak, 2012) that is experienced as aversive (Proudfit, Inzlicht, & Mennin, 2012). Interestingly, both dispositional and experimentally induced acceptance toward errors is associated with larger ERNs and improved self-control. In a recent study, meditators reported greater emotional acceptance, larger ERNs, and fewer Stroop errors compared to non-meditators (Teper & Inzlicht, 2013). Critically, acceptance was also positively correlated with ERN amplitudes, and it mediated the relationship between hours of meditation and Stroop error rate such that the greater emotional acceptance predicted better self-control. These findings are consistent with another study that explicitly manipulated acceptance and openness to threat, where participants who engaged in a self-affirmation exercise had larger ERNs and fewer errors in a self-control task than participants who engaged in a non-affirming exercise (Legault, Al-Khindi, & Inzlicht, 2012).

How can acceptance account for larger neural responses and improved performance on self-control tasks? Because mindfulness practices foster openness and non-judgement towards primary affective cues, meditators may experience the affective consequences of errors more keenly and purely, permitting negative affect to deploy self-control with greater efficiency. By being more accepting of the "pang" of negative affect at the moment of the error, one affords it a higher chance of disrupting routine behaviour, capturing attention, and motivating compensatory processes that prevent its future reoccurrence.

The complementarity of awareness and acceptance

We believe that, far from serving as merely independent and sequential contributors to self-control, both facets of mindfulness work jointly to enhance negative affect's instrumental relationship with self-control (Teper et al., 2013). Both awareness and acceptance seem to be involved in earlier and later stages of the affect-control relationship, and it may be that the order of their effects is contextual.

In one direction, interoceptive awareness is likely involved in the early detection and recognition of affective cues from goal conflicts, while a mindset of non-judgemental acceptance then allows such cues to unfold in the experiential field without cognitive intrusion. For example, if a person who wants to manage their anger at work is attuned to their internal experiences, they will be more likely to notice incipient affective cues (e.g. "pangs" of anxiety or guilt) indicating that their present behaviour is socially inappropriate. If that person is also accepting and open towards their primary affective experiences, then those affective cues will have a higher likelihood of recruiting self-control without interference from other moment-to-moment thoughts or appraisals. In such a case, awareness enables the recognition of affective cues that may be subtle, while acceptance allows those cues to retain their instrumental quality against processes capable of diminishing it.

In the other direction, a cultivated acceptance and openness to primary experiences may strengthen and intensify the affective cues that accompany goal conflicts, affording them greater visibility among the assortment of sensations, emotions, and thoughts present in the experiential field. When this is combined with a cultivated interoceptive awareness, a person trying to control their anger may have greater leverage in spontaneously shifting their conscious attention towards the strong affective cues indicating the need for self-control. In this case, acceptance amplifies the affective cues from goal conflicts, while awareness increases the chance that those amplified cues will capture attention.

Our model does not specify which of these descriptions is more plausible; they are not mutually exclusive, so it is even possible that both are correct. Importantly, both views highlight the complementary relationship between awareness and acceptance, and imply that the cultivation of only one component is less likely to facilitate self-control.

Conclusions and future directions

In this chapter, we have sketched a basic model that outlines the facilitative effect of mindfulness on self-control. When we view self-control as a fundamentally emotional process, it follows that movers of emotion – like mindfulness – will influence it. Evidence suggests that the interoceptive awareness and non-judgemental acceptance fostered by mindfulness practice can moderate response to conflict-related affect, or moderate conflict-related affect itself. Importantly, our model goes beyond the conventional perspective that mindfulness improves behavioural outcomes primarily through attenuating maladaptive thought processes or negative emotions over time. On the contrary, we believe that it can also heighten our sensitivity to rapid and transient negative emotions, allowing them to mobilize self-control processes that realign our behaviour with our goals.

However, our model leaves a number of questions about mindfulness, affect, and self-control unanswered. For instance, does non-judgemental acceptance primarily function to enhance affective cues, or primarily function to protect those cues from cognitive obfuscations? Do the contributions of awareness and acceptance vary based on context or their degree of cultivation? How do awareness and acceptance relate to the positive and rewarding aspects of unhealthy stimuli that cause goal conflicts in the first place? Future studies may begin to answer these questions by investigating the temporal dynamics of acceptance and awareness during circumstances that require self-control. This could be ideally accomplished in longitudinal designs that combine clinical, physiological, and experience sampling methods.

Our theoretical approach may also prove fruitful for examining the therapeutic effects of awareness and acceptance on patients with characteristically poor self-control. Is merely awareness or merely acceptance sufficient for the best therapeutic outcomes, or are both truly necessary for long-lasting change? Several studies that have investigated the effects of Acceptance Commitment Therapy on self-control–related disorders, such as alcohol abuse (Heffner, Eifert, Parker, Hernandez, & Sperry, 2003) and eating pathologies (Juarascio, Forman, & Herbert, 2010), suggest that at least in some cases, acceptance alone may be sufficient for self-control improvement. From a theoretic standpoint, however, practitioners have warned against cultivating either skill set in isolation. In psychotherapy, for instance, awareness without acceptance may leave the patient unequipped to deal appropriately with negative affect (see Cardaciotto et al., 2008). Cultivating acceptance without awareness, conversely, may foster a complacency of emotional discomfort (Siegel, Germer, & Olendzki, 2009). In sum, a more thorough exploration of the independent pathways from awareness and acceptance to self-control is needed in both the experimental and clinical sciences before moving forward.

References

Baer, R. A., Smith, G. T., & Allen, K. B. (2004). Assessment of mindfulness by self-report: The Kentucky Inventory of mindfulness skills. *Assessment, 11*(3), 191–206.

Bailey, K., Bartholow, B. D., Saults, J. S., & Lust, S. A. (2014). Give me just a little more time: Effects of alcohol on the failure and recovery of cognitive control. *Journal of Abnormal Psychology, 123*(1), 152–167.

Barrett, L. F., Gross, J., Christensen, T. C., & Benvenuto, M. (2001). Knowing what you're feeling and knowing what to do about it: Mapping the relation between emotion differentiation and emotion regulation. *Cognition & Emotion, 15*(6), 713–724.

Bartholow, B. D., Henry, E. A., Lust, S. A., Saults, J. S., & Wood, P. K. (2012). Alcohol effects on performance monitoring and adjustment: Affect modulation and impairment of evaluative cognitive control. *Journal of Abnormal Psychology, 121*(1), 173.

Botvinick, M. M., Braver, T. S., Barch, D. M., Carter, C. S., & Cohen, J. D. (2001). Conflict monitoring and cognitive control. *Psychological Review, 108*(3), 624–652.

Bowen, S., Witkiewitz, K., Dillworth, T. M., Chawla, N., Simpson, T. L., Ostafin, B. D., . . . Marlatt, G. A. (2006). Mindfulness meditation and substance use in an incarcerated population. *Psychology of Addictive Behaviors, 20*(3), 343–347.

Brown, K. W., & Ryan, R. M. (2003). The benefits of being present: Mindfulness and its role in psychological well-being. *Journal of Personality and Social Psychology, 84*(4), 822.

Cardaciotto, L., Herbert, J. D., Forman, E. M., Moitra, E., & Farrow, V. (2008). The assessment of present-moment awareness and acceptance: The Philadelphia Mindfulness Scale. *Assessment, 15*(2), 204–223.

Carver, C. S., & Scheier, M. F. (1998). *On the self-regulation of behavior.* Cambridge: Cambridge University Press.

Chan, D., & Woollacott, M. (2007). Effects of level of meditation experience on attentional focus: Is the efficiency of executive or orientation networks improved? *The Journal of Alternative and Complementary Medicine, 13*(6), 651–658.

Chiesa, A., & Serretti, A. (2014). Are mindfulness-based interventions effective for substance use disorders? A systematic review of the evidence. *Substance Use & Misuse, 49*(5), 492–512.

Daubenmier, J., Sze, J., Kerr, C. E., Kemeny, M. E., & Mehling, W. (2013). Follow your breath: Respiratory interoceptive accuracy in experienced meditators. *Psychophysiology, 50*(8), 777–789.

Davidson, R. J., & Kaszniak, A. W. (2015). Conceptual and methodological issues in research on mindfulness and meditation. *American Psychologist, 70*(7), 581–592.

Deikman, A. J. (1996). "I" = awareness. *Journal of Consciousness Studies, 3*, 350–356.

Donohue, K. F., Curtin, J. J., Patrick, C. J., & Lang, A. R. (2007). Intoxication level and emotional response. *Emotion, 7*(1), 103–112.

Easdon, C., Izenberg, A., Armilio, M. L., Yu, H., & Alain, C. (2005). Alcohol consumption impairs stimulus- and error-related processing during a Go/No-Go Task. *Cognitive Brain Research, 25*(3), 873–883.

Ehlers, A., & Breuer, P. (1992). Increased cardiac awareness in panic disorder. *Journal of Abnormal Psychology, 101*(3), 371.

Ehlers, A., & Breuer, P. (1996). How good are patients with panic disorder at perceiving their heartbeats? *Biological Psychology, 42*(1), 165–182.

Elwafi, H. M., Witkiewitz, K., Mallik, S., Thornhill, T. A., IV, & Brewer, J. A. (2013). Mindfulness training for smoking cessation: Moderation of the relationship between craving and cigarette use. *Drug and Alcohol Dependence, 130*(1–3), 222–229.

Erbas, Y., Ceulemans, E., Lee Pe, M., Koval, P., & Kuppens, P. (2014). Negative emotion differentiation: Its personality and well-being correlates and a comparison of different assessment methods. *Cognition and Emotion, 28*(7), 1196–1213.

Fan, J., McCandliss, B. D., Sommer, T., Raz, A., & Posner, M. I. (2002). Testing the efficiency and independence of attentional networks. *Journal of Cognitive Neuroscience, 14*(3), 340–347.

Farb, N. A. S., Daubenmier, J., Price, C. J., Gard, T., Kerr, C., Dunn, B. D., . . . Mehling, W. E. (2015). Interoception, contemplative practice, and health. *Frontiers in Psychology, 6*, 763.

Farb, N. A. S., Segal, Z. V., & Anderson, A. K. (2013). Mindfulness meditation training alters cortical representations of interoceptive attention. *Social Cognitive and Affective Neuroscience, 8*(1), 15–26.

Farb, N. A. S., Segal, Z. V., Mayberg, H., Bean, J., McKeon, D., Fatima, Z., & Anderson, A. K. (2007). Attending to the present: Mindfulness meditation reveals distinct neural modes of self-reference. *Social Cognitive and Affective Neuroscience, 2*(4), 313–322.

Fox, K. C. R., Zakarauskas, P., Dixon, M., Ellamil, M., Thompson, E., & Christoff, K. (2012). Meditation experience predicts introspective accuracy. *PLoS ONE, 7*(9), e45370.

Frijda, N. H. (1988). The laws of emotion. *American Psychologist, 43*(5), 349–358. doi:10.1037/0003-066x.43.5.349

Fujita, K. (2011). On conceptualizing self-control as more than the effortful inhibition of impulses. *Personality and Social Psychology Review, 15*(4), 352–366.

Gard, T., Hölzel, B. K., Sack, A. T., Hempel, H., Lazar, S. W., Vaitl, D., & Ott, U. (2012). Pain attenuation through mindfulness is associated with decreased cognitive control and increased sensory processing in the brain. *Cerebral Cortex, 22*(11), 2692–2702.

Gehring, W. J., Goss, B., Coles, M. G. H., Meyer, D. E., & Donchin, E. (1993). A neural system for error detection and compensation. *Psychological Science, 4*(6), 385–390.

Grant, J. A., Courtemanche, J., & Rainville, P. (2011). A non-elaborative mental stance and decoupling of executive and pain-related cortices predicts low pain sensitivity in Zen meditators. *Pain, 152*(1), 150–156.

Gray, J. A., & McNaughton, N. (2000). *The neuropsychology of anxiety: An enquiry into the functions of the septo-hippocampal system.* Oxford: Oxford University Press.

Gross, J. J. (1998). The emerging field of emotion regulation: An integrative review. *Review of General Psychology, 2*(3), 271–299.

Hajcak, G., & Foti, D. (2008). Errors are aversive defensive motivation and the error-related negativity. *Psychological Science, 19*(2), 103–108.

Hart, W. (2011). *The art of living: Vipassana meditation as taught by S. N. Goenka.* Onalaska, WA: Pariyatti.

Hayes, S. C. (1994). Content, context, and the types of psychological acceptance. In S. C. Hayes, N. S. Jacobsen, V. M. Follette, & M. J. Dougher (Eds.), *Acceptance & change: Content and context in psychotherapy* (pp. 13–32). Reno, NV: Context Press.

Heffner, M., Eifert, G. H., Parker, B. T., Hernandez, D. H., & Sperry, J. A. (2003). Valued directions: Acceptance and commitment therapy in the treatment of alcohol dependence. *Cognitive and Behavioral Practice, 10*(4), 378–383.

Hill, C. L. M., & Updegraff, J. A. (2012). Mindfulness and its relationship to emotional regulation. *Emotion, 12*, 81–90.

Hofmann, W., Friese, M., & Strack, F. (2009). Impulse and self-control from a dual-systems perspective. *Perspectives on Psychological Science, 4*(2), 162–176.

Holroyd, C. B., & Coles, M. G. H. (2002). The neural basis of human error processing: Reinforcement learning, dopamine, and the error-related negativity. *Psychological Review, 109*(4), 679–709.

Inzlicht, M., Bartholow, B. D., & Hirsh, J. B. (2015). Emotional foundations of cognitive control. *Trends in Cognitive Sciences, 19*(3), 126–132.

Jha, A. P., Krompinger, J., & Baime, M. J. (2007). Mindfulness training modifies subsystems of attention. *Cognitive, Affective, & Behavioral Neuroscience, 7*(2), 109–119.

Juarascio, A. S., Forman, E. M., & Herbert, J. D. (2010). Acceptance and commitment therapy versus cognitive therapy for the treatment of comorbid eating pathology. *Behavior Modification, 34*(2), 175–190.

Kabat-Zinn, J. (1994). *Wherever you go, there you are: Mindfulness meditation in everyday life.* New York: Hyperion.

Lee, N. K., Greely, J., & Oei, T. P. (1999). The relationship of positive and negative alcohol expectancies to patterns of consumption of alcohol in social drinkers. *Addictive Behaviors, 24*(3), 359–369.

Legault, L., Al-Khindi, T., & Inzlicht, M. (2012). Preserving integrity in the face of performance threat: Self-affirmation enhances neurophysiological responsiveness to errors. *Psychological Science, 23*(12), 1455–1460.

Levenson, R. W., Sher, K. J., Grossman, L. M., Newman, J., & Newlin, D. B. (1980). Alcohol and stress response dampening: Pharmacological effects, expectancy, and tension reduction. *Journal of Abnormal Psychology, 89*(4), 528.

Levinson, D. B., Stoll, E. L., Kindy, S. D., Merry, H. L., & Davidson, R. J. (2014). A mind you can count on: Validating breath counting as a behavioral measure of mindfulness. *Frontiers in Psychology, 5*(1202), 1–10.

Marlatt, G. A., & Kristeller, J. L. (1999). Mindfulness and meditation. In W. R. Miller (Ed.), *Integrating spirituality into treatment* (pp. 67–84). Washington, DC: American Psychological Association.

McCracken, L. M. (1997). "Attention" to pain in persons with chronic pain: A behavioral approach. *Behavior Therapy, 28*(2), 271–284.

Metcalfe, J., & Mischel, W. (1999). A hot/cool-system analysis of delay of gratification: Dynamics of willpower. *Psychological Review, 106*(1), 3–19.

Miyake, A., & Friedman, N. P. (2012). The nature and organization of individual differences in executive functions: Four general conclusions. *Current Directions in Psychological Science, 21*(1), 8–14.

Miyake, A., Friedman, N. P., Emerson, M. J., Witzki, A. H., Howerter, A., & Wager, T. D. (2000). The unity and diversity of executive functions and their contributions to complex "frontal lobe" tasks: A latent variable analysis. *Cognitive psychology, 41*(1), 49–100.

Moore, A., & Malinowski, P. (2009). Meditation, mindfulness and cognitive flexibility. *Conscious Cognition, 18*(1), 176–186.

Nielsen, L., & Kaszniak, A. W. (2006). Awareness of subtle emotional feelings: A comparison of long-term meditators and nonmeditators. *Emotion, 6*(3), 392–405.

Ochsner, K., & Gross, J. (2005). The cognitive control of emotion. *Trends in Cognitive Sciences, 9*(5), 242–249.

Parrott, W. G., & Schulkin, J. (1993). Neuropsychology and the cognitive nature of the emotions. *Cognition & Emotion, 7*(1), 43–59.

Perkins, A. M., Ettinger, U., Davis, R., Foster, R., Williams, S. C., & Corr, P. J. (2009). Effects of lorazepam and citalopram on human defensive reactions: Ethopharmacological differentiation of fear and anxiety. *The Journal of Neuroscience, 29*(40), 12617–12624.

Perkins, A. M., Ettinger, U., Weaver, K., Schmechtig, A., Schrantee, A., Morrison, P. D., . . . Corr, P. J. (2013). Advancing the defensive explanation for anxiety disorders: Lorazepam effects on human defense are systematically modulated by personality and threat-type. *Translational Psychiatry, 3*(4), e246.

Pessoa, L. (2008). On the relationship between emotion and cognition. *Nature Reviews Neuroscience, 9*(2), 148–158.

Proudfit, G. H., Inzlicht, M., & Mennin, D. S. (2012). Anxiety and error monitoring: The importance of motivation and emotion. *Frontiers in Human Neuroscience, 7,* 636–644.

Ridderinkhof, K. R., de Vlugt, Y., Bramlage, A., Spaan, M., Elton, M., Snel, J., & Band, G. P. (2002). Alcohol consumption impairs detection of performance errors in mediofrontal cortex. *Science, 298*(5601), 2209–2211.

Roemer, L., & Orsillo, S. M. (2003). Mindfulness: A promising intervention strategy in need of further study. *Clinical Psychology: Science and Practice, 10*(2), 172–178.

Russell, J. A. (2003). Core affect and the psychological construction of emotion. *Psychological Review, 110*(1), 145–172.

Russell, J. A., & Barrett, L. F. (1999). Core affect, prototypical emotional episodes, and other things called emotion: Dissecting the elephant. *Journal of Personality and Social Psychology, 76*(5), 805–819.

Saunders, B., Milyavskaya, M., & Inzlicht, M. (2015). Variation in cognitive control as emotion regulation. *Psychological Inquiry, 26*(1), 108–115.

Schachter, S., & Singer, J. (1962). Cognitive, social, and physiological determinants of emotional state. *Psychological Review, 69*(5), 379–399.

Siegel, R. D., Germer, C. K., & Olendzki, A. (2009). Mindfulness: What is it? Where did it come from? In F. Didonna (Ed.), *Clinical handbook of mindfulness* (pp. 17–35). New York: Springer.

Stark, R., Walter, B., Schienle, A., & Vaitl, D. (2005). Psychophysiological correlates of disgust and disgust sensitivity. *Journal of Psychophysiology, 19*(1), 50–60.

Tang, Y. Y., Ma, Y., Wang, J., Fan, Y., Feng, S., Lu, Q., . . . Posner, M. I. (2007). Short-term meditation training improves attention and self-regulation. *Proceedings of the National Academy of Sciences, 104*(43), 17152–17156.

Tang, Y. Y., Tang, R., & Posner, M. I. (2013). Brief meditation training induces smoking reduction. *Proceedings of the National Academy Sciences, 110*(34), 13971–13975.

Teper, R., & Inzlicht, M. (2013). Meditation, mindfulness and executive control: The importance of emotional acceptance and brain-based performance monitoring. *Social Cognitive and Affective Neuroscience, 8*(1), 85–92.

Van den Hurk, P. A. M., Janssen, B. H., Giommi, F., Barendregt, H. P., & Gielen, S. C. (2010). Mindfulness meditation associated with alterations in bottom-up processing: Psychophysiological evidence for reduced reactivity. *International Journal of Psychophysiology, 78*(2), 151–157.

Vohs, K. D., & Baumeister, R. F. (2011). Understanding self-regulation: An introduction. In K. Vohs & R. Baumeister (Eds.), *Handbook of self-regulation: Research, theory, and applications* (pp. 1–9). New York: Guilford Press.

Vrana, S. R. (1993). The psychophysiology of disgust: Differentiating negative emotional contexts with facial EMG. *Psychophysiology, 30*(3), 279–286.

Weinberg, A., Riesel, A., & Hajcak, G. (2012). Integrating multiple perspectives on error-related brain activity: The ERN as a neural indicator of trait defensive reactivity. *Motivation and Emotion, 36*(1), 84–100.

Wenk-Sormaz, H. (2005). Meditation can reduce habitual responding. *Alternative Therapies in Health and Medicine, 11*(2), 42.

Yeung, N., Ralph, J., & Nieuwenhuis, S. (2007). Drink alcohol and dim the lights: The impact of cognitive deficits on medial frontal cortex function. *Cognitive, Affective, & Behavioral Neuroscience, 7*(4), 347–355.

6

MINDFULNESS, EMOTION REGULATION, AND SOCIAL THREAT

Jerry Slutsky, Hayley Rahl, Emily K. Lindsay, and J. David Creswell

Mindfulness (and mindfulness training interventions) are consistently and robustly linked with alterations in markers of emotional experience (Chambers, Gullone, & Allen, 2009), leading many researchers in social psychology and related fields to posit that emotion regulation processes may be a key mechanism underlying mindfulness outcomes (Brown, Ryan, & Creswell, 2007; Hölzel et al., 2011). To describe just a few of these effects, mindfulness training interventions have been shown to decrease anxiety for those with social/generalized anxiety disorder, prevent depressive relapse in at-risk patients, and improve mood in healthy populations (Desrosiers, Vine, Klemanski, & Nolen-Hoeksema, 2013; Goldin & Gross, 2010; Hölzel et al., 2013; Kuyken et al., 2008; Quaglia, Brown, Lindsay, Creswell, & Goodman, 2014). In this chapter we consider this important topic of mindfulness and emotion regulation, first summarizing a comprehensive contemporary model of emotion regulation processes (Gross, 1998) and then discussing how mindfulness may impact these emotion regulation processes. Specifically, we will unpack an account positing that mindfulness affects attentional deployment (how one attends to emotional stimuli), which in turn impacts emotion processing and emotion-related responses over time. We conclude the chapter with a consideration of how these mindfulness-emotion regulation effects may impact a broad range of social threat responses of relevance to social psychology.

What is emotion regulation and how might mindfulness impact it?

Emotions can be beneficial when they facilitate social interactions, bring our attention to key features of the environment, and enhance our ability to remember specific events. However, emotions can also be a detriment to our social interactions, attention, and memory when they are the wrong type, intensity, or duration, or when we cannot regulate them effectively to meet the demands of a situation. In his popular model of emotion regulation, Gross (1998) delineates the processes that must occur to successfully regulate one's emotions over time, moving from situation selection to situation modification, attentional deployment, cognitive change, and response modulation. According to the model, one may employ *situation selection* by approaching or avoiding certain people, places, or objects. Once exposed to an emotional situation, one can then modify the situation so as to alter its emotional impact (termed *situation modification*). Next, *attentional deployment* refers to which aspect of a situation a person focuses on. A common form of attentional deployment is distraction, which focuses attention on another aspect of the situation or away from the situation altogether. By contrast, to preview an idea we develop in this chapter, initial studies suggest that mindful individuals deploy their attention towards emotional stimuli (Lebois et al., 2015; Teper & Inzlicht, 2013; Vago & Nakamura, 2011). *Cognitive change* refers to modifying how one appraises a situation so as to alter its emotional significance. Last, *response modulation* pertains to directly influencing physiological, experiential, or behavioural responding. This emotion regulation process has been applied to a broad range of outcomes, such as coping with anxiety or pain (see recent reviews: Gross, 2015; Webb, Miles, & Sheeran, 2012).

How might mindfulness alter these emotion regulation processes? Mindfulness of an emotional experience involves recognizing that an emotion is present, allowing it to be there, and investigating the ongoing qualities of this emotion without judgement (e.g. body sensations, thoughts, images, and reactions). Consider the scenario of tripping and falling in a cafeteria, spilling a tray of food in front of one's peers. An individual with high levels of trait mindfulness (as measured by a number of self-report measures; Quaglia et al., 2014), or someone who has developed mindfulness through a mindfulness training program (e.g. the 8-week Mindfulness-Based Stress Reduction program), might turn his or her attention to rapidly rising and intense feelings of embarrassment, notice body sensations and thoughts from this social blunder, and maintain an open and accepting attentional stance towards these responses, instead of suppressing these feelings or turning to angry self-directed thoughts. By attending to one's emotional experience with acceptance ('mindful attention'), one is able to stay in contact with feelings of embarrassment and associated body states, perhaps noticing that they dwindle to baseline levels. As this scenario illustrates, mindfulness may foster greater attention and acceptance towards one's emotional experience, and subsequently alter one's emotional responses.

In this scenario and, we propose, in many other daily life emotion-generating experiences, mindfulness first intervenes during the attentional deployment stage when one orients towards stimuli in an accepting manner (Brown & Ryan, 2003; Kabat-Zinn & Hanh, 2009). Furthermore, we believe that the impact of mindfulness on attentional deployment feeds forward to affect each of the following emotion regulation stages, resulting in increased availability and flexibility of cognitive change strategies (i.e. regulatory flexibility) and more effective response modulation, all of which may feed back to affect future situation selection and modification. Figure 6.1 depicts how mindfulness putatively affects the emotion regulation process.

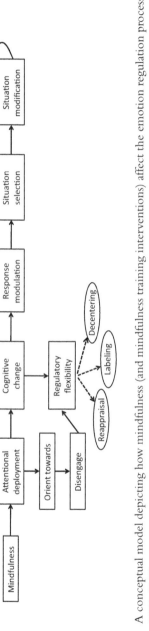

FIGURE 6.1 A conceptual model depicting how mindfulness (and mindfulness training interventions) affect the emotion regulation process (Gross, 1998, 2015)

Mindfulness and attentional deployment: Early attention to threat

Attentional deployment is the emotion regulation process of directing attention toward or away from specific stimuli in order to influence emotional responding. When confronted with a threatening situation, such as giving a presentation or being interviewed for a job, one may either deploy attention towards feelings of stress and anxiety or away from them (Gross, 2015). We consider the available empirical evidence linking mindfulness and emotion regulation processes with threat stimuli to suggest that mindfulness can influence attentional deployment as early as within a few hundred milliseconds (ms) (Brown, Goodman, & Inzlicht, 2013; Teper & Inzlicht, 2013; Vago & Nakamura, 2011). For example, after 8 weeks of mindfulness training, fibromyalgia patients oriented their attention more toward pain-related word threats, an effect that was observed 100ms after presentation of the threat stimulus (Vago & Nakamura, 2011). Furthermore, when threat stimuli were displayed for 500ms, participants in the mindfulness training condition (relative to the age-matched controls) were faster to disengage their attention from threat. This suggests that mindfulness training reduces both avoidance of threat and elaborative processing of threat. In another study, long-term meditators oriented towards error commission on the Stroop task; compared to non-meditators, they showed a greater neurophysiological response at 100ms as measured using error-related negativity, an event-related potential (ERP) (Teper & Inzlicht, 2013). The meditators also reported higher levels of acceptance and made fewer errors, providing evidence that early attentional deployment toward emotional stimuli may improve cognitive processing outcomes (see also Elkins-Brown, Teper, & Inzlicht, Chapter 5 in this volume).

In recent work, we describe the dissociable and interactive effects of the two basic components of mindfulness: attention monitoring and acceptance (Lindsay & Creswell, 2017). We suggest that training one's attention to monitor present-moment experience, the 'monitoring' component of mindfulness, may be an important mechanism that enhances orienting towards momentary emotional stimuli very early in the attention process (~100ms). Notably, early effects on the attention network (Attention Network Task) have been observed behaviourally in several mindfulness training studies, such that individuals showed improvements in conflict monitoring after brief, 5-day training (Tang et al., 2007), and improvements in orienting towards spatial cues after 8-week training (Jha, Krompinger, & Baime, 2007).

Not only is there initial evidence that mindfulness fosters early attention orienting to threat, but studies have suggested that mindfulness can modulate attentional responses after initial orienting. Prior work provides evidence that high levels of trait mindfulness are associated with a lower neurophysiological response (lower amplitudes during late positive potential, an ERP) to threat (and pleasant images) at 400–500ms (Brown et al., 2013). Acceptance may be key in facilitating disengagement with emotional stimuli. Mindful individuals bring a non-judgemental acceptance to moment-by-moment experiences, which may allow them to 'let go' from any valence attached with the emotional experience as they continue to attend to new arising present-moment experiences.

In summary, initial studies have shown that mindfulness aids in orienting towards negative stimuli at ~100ms, and that mindfulness assists in modulating one's attentional response to negative stimuli at ~500ms (Brown et al., 2013; Teper & Inzlicht, 2013; Vago & Nakamura, 2011). Prior to this important work, there was very little consideration about how mindfulness might impact early attention processes (within the first half-second); our review of these initial studies suggests that mindfulness may have a number of important modulatory roles. First, mindfulness facilitates immediate engagement and orienting towards emotion-relevant information in the first ~100ms, and subsequent disengagement around 400–500ms. We still know little about the nature and mechanisms of how mindfulness might have such early attention effects (though we have offered initial theorizing about attention monitoring and acceptance playing important roles in these early attention deployment effects). Moreover, few studies have investigated the effects of mindfulness on early attention to positive stimuli (Brown et al., 2013). However, because attention monitoring presumably facilitates engagement with momentary stimuli, and acceptance allows for disengagement with these stimuli, we suspect that mindfulness will similarly modulate attention to positive and negative stimuli. In the next section, we discuss the implications of these early attentional modulations for subsequent cognitive change processes (cf. Gross, 1998).

Mindfulness and cognitive change

Our mindfulness-emotion regulation model (see Figure 6.1) illustrates the impact of mindfulness on attentional deployment (engaging and then disengaging with emotional stimuli) and subsequent effects on downstream emotion regulation processes, including cognitive change (Gross, 1998). Cognitive change consists of modifying appraisals of an emotion-eliciting stimulus (Gross, 2015), and there is evidence that mindfulness enhances cognitive change strategies, including affect labelling and cognitive reappraisal (Creswell, Way, Eisenberger, & Lieberman, 2007; Hölzel et al., 2013; Modinos, Ormel, & Aleman, 2010). One possible explanation that we further develop in this chapter attributes the mindful practice of monitoring ongoing emotional responses through an accepting lens towards reducing attachment and/or reactions to initial appraisals of emotion-eliciting stimuli. We propose that this effect enhances cognitive change by fostering greater regulatory flexibility (cf. Bonanno & Burton, 2013).

Recall the earlier example of feeling embarrassment after spilling food in the cafeteria. One set of maladaptive cognitive emotion regulation strategies that might occur in this situation include *suppression* of one's feelings or *rumination* on the embarrassment of making a mistake in front of one's peers. These strategies are associated with increased risk for mood disorders, such as depression and anxiety (Aldao & Nolen-Hoeksema, 2010). Mindful individuals may instead be able to orient towards and acknowledge initial feelings of embarrassment and fear and then accept these feelings as fleeting reactions, leaving room to respond in a variety of adaptive ways. One available adaptive response is positive reappraisal, or the process of reconstructing stressful events as benign, beneficial, and/or meaningful (Garland, Gaylord, & Park, 2009). In this particular scenario, positive reappraisal may facilitate viewing the scenario as an opportunity to make light of the situation and as a funny story to share. Mindfulness might also lead to the implementation of other adaptive strategies, such as decentering. In this scenario, decentering may allow one to broaden attention to include neutral, present-moment experiences of bodily sensations and focus on the sights and sounds of the cafeteria while the feelings of embarrassment dissipate.

Additional downstream emotion regulation processes that may be impacted by the effects of mindfulness on attentional deployment include the feedback and repertoire components of emotion regulation flexibility (Bonanno & Burton, 2013). *Feedback* is described as being able to notice when a regulatory strategy is not effective, and *repertoire* refers to utilizing a range of regulatory strategies that can accommodate the contextual demands (Bonanno & Burton, 2013). Because mindfulness improves attention orienting (e.g. Vago & Nakamura, 2011), mindful individuals might also more quickly notice when a regulatory strategy is ineffective and disengage from that strategy, thus enhancing feedback. Although the speed with which mindful individuals are able to identify ineffective strategies and choose a more effective regulatory strategy has not yet been studied (to our knowledge), mindfulness has been linked with more effective use of a range of regulatory strategies. Specifically, previous studies show that individuals higher in dispositional mindfulness show greater neural regulatory responses when asked to use affect labelling or cognitive reappraisal strategies (Brown et al., 2007; Garland et al., 2009; Hölzel et al., 2011; Modinos et al., 2010). Decentering, a regulatory strategy described earlier in this section, is the process of distancing the self from present experience by perceiving thoughts, feelings, and reactions as impermanent patterns of mental activity rather than as true representations of the self, and may facilitate beneficial effects of mindfulness on affective and social outcomes (Fresco et al., 2007; Hayes-Skelton & Graham, 2013; Lebois et al., 2015). Previous research has found a link between mindfulness, decentering, and decreased negative reactivity, in that participants assigned to a mindful breathing exercise (as compared to loving-kindness meditation and progressive muscle relaxation) reported greater levels of decentering (Toronto Mindfulness Scale, decentering subscale), as well as less frequent repetitive thoughts and reduced negative reactivity to those thoughts (Feldman, Greeson, & Senville, 2010). Previous research also suggests that mindfulness improves affective outcomes through the mechanism of decentering, including social anxiety and worry (Hayes-Skelton & Graham, 2013; Hoge et al., 2013). Mindfulness and decentering may reduce negative affect by altering the objectivity with which individuals view themselves and their symptoms (Farb et al., 2007).

In this section we have provided initial considerations of the role of mindfulness in emotion regulation processes, specifically cognitive change, with a focus on mindfulness increasing access to a broader range of cognitive change strategies and more flexible use of these strategies – which reflects greater regulatory flexibility (Bonanno & Burton, 2013). We also briefly highlighted initial evidence that mindfulness facilitates effective use of cognitive change strategies (e.g. affect labelling, reappraisal, decentering) (Creswell et al., 2007; Garland et al., 2009; Hayes-Skelton & Graham, 2013; Lebois et al., 2015; Modinos et al., 2010). We note that there is no work (to our knowledge) that directly tests whether mindfulness increases the number of regulatory strategies in one's repertoire or promotes more appropriate selection among strategies, which are important directions for future research. It may also be the case that mindfulness can promote strategic use of regulatory strategies that are sometimes considered maladaptive, such as distraction or suppression.

Selecting and utilizing regulatory strategies that are appropriate for the given situation can improve the regulation of emotion and subsequent response to emotion (Gross, 2015). In the next section, we consider evidence that explains how mindfulness might influence the selection of appropriate regulatory strategies and how this affects coping responses to stress.

Mindfulness and response modulation

If mindfulness alters the emotion regulation processes of attentional deployment and cognitive change, these alterations may affect downstream coping with an emotional situation (termed 'response modulation' by Gross, 1998). Common ways that people respond to emotionally evocative situations include the use of alcohol, drugs, food, humour, social and religious support, and emotional suppression in order to alter their feeling states (Carver, Scheier, & Weintraub, 1989). In contrast, mindfulness may turn down emotional reactivity (e.g. Arch & Craske, 2010; Broderick, 2005) and increase approach-oriented coping efforts (Weinstein, Brown, & Ryan, 2009). Research suggests that mindfulness helps individuals view demanding situations as less threatening or stressful, which facilitates more adaptive coping (Weinstein et al., 2009). Mindful individuals use fewer avoidance-oriented strategies and more approach-oriented coping strategies, and this increased use of adaptive strategies explains reductions in self-reported anxiety and improvements in well-being (Weinstein et al., 2009). We speculate that mindfulness may facilitate selection of adaptive coping strategies by buffering one's response to acute stress (perhaps through early reappraisal) and accelerating the recovery from stress (perhaps through monitoring thoughts, emotions, and sensations with acceptance), such that one does not resort to maladaptive strategies in order to placate heightened feelings of stress. Indeed, we and others have found that mindfulness buffers psychological and biological responses to acute stress (Brown, Weinstein, & Creswell, 2012; Creswell, Pacilio, Lindsay, & Brown, 2014; Nyklíček, Dijksman, Lenders, Fonteijn, & Koolen, 2014; for a review, see Creswell & Lindsay, 2014), suggesting that mindfulness may foster improved coping with stress. Furthermore, prior work provides evidence that individuals who underwent an 8-week mindfulness training reported lower levels of anxiety in the first few minutes of recovery from the

Trier Social Stress Test (a social evaluative stress task) compared to a waitlist control group, suggesting that mindfulness may accelerate recovery from stress and facilitate a return to baseline levels (Britton, Shahar, Szepsenwol, & Jacobs, 2012).

We have provided initial theory and evidence suggesting that mindfulness may facilitate response modulation via modulation of coping responses to stress. In particular, mindfulness has been shown to alter stress appraisals by decreasing perception of threat, which may in turn foster use of approach-oriented coping strategies (Weinstein et al., 2009). Little research (to our surprise) has examined how mindfulness alters response modulation and coping responses to stress in healthy individuals or those who are at-risk (e.g. mood and stress-related disorders).

Mindfulness and situation selection/modification

Sometimes in anticipation of an emotional situation, we take initiative to regulate its emotional impact by avoiding or modifying the situation (Gross, 1998). Before we allow an argument with a spouse or child to escalate, we take a break from the disagreement and walk outside to cool down. Or, when watching a scary movie and a violent scene is expected to appear, we turn the volume down or look away to avoid becoming too frightened. Walking away from an argument is an example of situation selection, or taking action to reduce the likelihood that undesirable emotions will arise (Gross, 2015). Muting a scary movie is an example of situation modification, as this action alters the situation in a way that changes its emotional impact (Gross, 2015). Although little work has examined this emotion regulation process, we speculate that mindfulness may have a role in modulating situation selection and modification. Previously discussed evidence suggests that mindfulness may foster an enhanced capacity to identify a negative situation and the cognitive flexibility to decide if one has the coping resources to manage the situation. It follows that a more mindful individual might show greater foresight to enter, leave, or modify the situation to preclude a negative affective response. An intriguing prediction from this account is that mindfulness may foster greater pro-active coping prior to stressful events (Aspinwall & Taylor, 1997), such that mindfulness training helps individuals see potential stressors on the horizon and avoid them entirely. Alternatively, if a stressor is likely, then mindfulness may facilitate efforts to marshal resources in ways that mitigate the impact of the stressor. Another alternative is that mindfulness might dissuade one from taking immediate action, instead bringing focus to accepting whatever occurs in the present moment.

Research is needed to clarify the effects of mindfulness (both trait and trained mindfulness) on situation selection and situation modification outcomes. There are many possibilities for future research on this topic. In the case of situation selection, it may be that mindfulness training interventions reduce the likelihood that substance-abusing individuals visit places that are likely to act as triggers for substance use (e.g. heavy drinkers/smokers visiting bars). In the case of situation modification, mindfulness training interventions may facilitate pro-active coping efforts by students in the weeks leading up to major exams (e.g. seeking help at office hours, forming study groups, daily exercise, regular sleep) in order to mitigate stress on exam day. Although mindfulness may encourage individuals to both approach and avoid stressful situations, we posit that mindful individuals are on average more likely to engage in these situations based on prior evidence showing that mindfulness can reduce one's perceptions of threat, and consequently reduce avoidance behaviour (Weinstein et al., 2009). Some theorists suggest that mindfulness facilitates addiction cessation and prevention by promoting acceptance, exposure, and openness (Heppner, Spears, Vidrine, & Wetter, 2015). Future research should clarify whether mindful individuals are avoiding or modifying stressful situations, engaging and coping with them, or a combination of these strategies.

Mindfulness, emotion regulation, and social threat

Social relationships provide some of the strongest emotional elicitors (Baumeister & Leary, 1995), and oftentimes high-quality social relationship functioning requires effective emotion regulation (Gross, 2002). Although initial work has investigated the effectiveness of mindfulness on buffering social threat (Barnes, Brown, Krusemark, Campbell, & Rogge, 2007; Brown et al., 2012; Creswell et al., 2014; Weinstein et al., 2009), the mechanisms linking emotion regulation processes, mindfulness, and social threat are still unclear. In this section, we consider the implications of our proposed mindfulness emotion regulation framework for social threat outcomes – a topic of relevance to social psychologists.

Emotion regulation strategies must be contextually appropriate in order to be considered adaptive responses to social threat. Social anxiety disorder and other psychiatric disorders often lead to inappropriate implementation of emotion regulation strategies, such as avoidance, and therefore the negative impact of these disorders might be lessened by training that increases use of contextually appropriate strategies (Jazaieri, Morrison, Goldin, & Gross, 2015). When the threat of social situations is exaggerated, situation selection (avoidance) may be used too frequently (Andersen & Teicher, 2008). In addition, when individuals exhibit biases towards threat (or attempt to avoid threat), as well as an inability to disengage from threat, they may be using attentional deployment in a maladaptive way. Mindfulness training may decrease the use of inappropriate emotion regulation strategies and improve social threat responses, perhaps through enhancing regulatory flexibility. Previous research has found that mindfulness may reduce social anxiety through the mechanism of decentering, and that cognitive reappraisal also reduces social anxiety through this pathway (Hayes-Skelton & Graham, 2013). This suggests that changing one's perspective to monitor experiences from a distance – rather than considering each experience in relation to oneself – may help to reduce anxiety in social situations (cf. Farb et al., 2007) and subsequently improve social and romantic relationships (Carson, Carson, Gil, & Baucom, 2004). Post-event processing, something that often exacerbates anxiety, may also be reduced by mindfulness and cognitive reappraisal, leading to improvements in affect (Baer, 2003; Brown et al., 2007; Hölzel et al., 2011; Shikatani, Antony, Kuo, & Cassin, 2014).

There are several initial studies suggesting that mindfulness (and mindfulness training interventions) can foster more effective use of emotion regulation strategies and buffer social threat responses. Recent work suggests that orienting towards threat with acceptance may help explain results that high dispositional mindfulness and self-esteem are predictors of lower levels of social anxiety (Rasmussen & Pidgeon, 2010). Other research measuring the effects of dispositional mindfulness on relationship conflict in romantic couples found that those with higher levels of dispositional mindfulness reported less emotional stress (lower post-conflict anxiety and anger-hostility levels) in response to a relationship conflict discussion with their romantic partner (Barnes et al., 2007; for a review, see Karremans, Schellekens, & Kappen, 2015; Karremans & Kappen, Chapter 8 in this volume). Notably, these effects were driven by the fact that participants who were high in dispositional mindfulness entered the conflict discussion with lower levels of emotional stress. This effect suggests that one's anxiety levels prior to a stressful event affect how one regulates emotions during the stressful event. Patterns of decreased reactivity and enhanced coping over time may feed back to influence the beginning stages of emotion regulation. Consistent with these findings, we have also shown that more mindful individuals have reduced psychological stress perceptions to the Trier Social Stress Test (TSST), a difficult social stress challenge task consisting of presenting a speech and performing difficult mental arithmetic in front of an evaluative audience (Brown et al., 2012; Creswell et al., 2014). Our model provides one possible interpretation for these findings, such that orienting towards a potential threat with acceptance during the attentional deployment stage can lead to lower threat appraisals, which buffers stress reactivity and leads to more adaptive forms of coping and faster physiological stress recovery.

Social exclusion, or, the process of being ostracized from social groups, is similar to other types of social threats previously discussed in that anxiety is produced when one's social needs are threatened – in this case, the need to belong (Baumeister & Tice, 1990). Mindfulness and social exclusion has yet to thoroughly be investigated; however, initial research found intriguing results in that a brief mindfulness induction was shown to expedite recovery from feelings of distress, after participants were excluded from a game of Cyberball (a virtual game of catch) (Molet, Macquet, Lefebvre, & Williams, 2013). These results suggest that mindfulness assists the process of minimizing time spent ruminating on past pain and returning one's attention to the present moment. As we previously mentioned, mindful individuals are more likely to perceive situations as less threatening and utilize an approach-oriented coping style (Weinstein et al., 2009). We believe that this would translate well to situations involving social exclusion, in that mindful individuals would be less paralyzed by distress experienced from ostracism, and more likely to take initiative to resolve the problem, such as confronting individuals committing ostracism and resolving the issues that may be at the root of the problem. Furthermore, mindfulness may buffer feelings of social exclusion in that it alters perceptions of loneliness, which might make one more comfortable with feeling alone (cf. Creswell et al., 2012).

Discussion

This chapter has considered the ways in which mindfulness might interact with the emotion regulation process (Gross, 1998). We have proposed that mindfulness may change the way one initially deploys attention and implements cognitive change strategies (which we have discussed as increasing one's regulatory flexibility). Further, we have considered how these alterations in attention deployment and cognitive change are likely to change subsequent response modulation, situation selection and situation modification. We aimed in this chapter to highlight initial promising mindfulness-emotion regulation links and evidence, while acknowledging that we still have very little empirical research on this topic. Our proposed model builds on previous theorizing and research on core components of emotion regulation (Gross, 1998, 2015) and regulatory flexibility (Bonanno & Burton, 2013), as well as our own theorizing about how mindfulness may fit as a core process in emotion regulation. We suspect, like others (Baer, 2003; Brown, Ryan, & Creswell, 2007; Hölzel et al., 2011), that emotion regulation processes may be an important underlying mechanism linking mindfulness with a broad range of outcomes in the growing body of literature – and we have briefly considered potential links with social threat outcomes.

There are still many open questions and considerations about mindfulness-emotion regulation links. Certainly, expertise is likely to alter mindfulness-emotion regulation dynamics – researchers have posited that expert meditators have an automatic accepting stance toward their experience ('non-appraisal'), such that they may not need to implement much in the way of cognitive change (Hölzel et al., 2011). In support of this hypothesis, when experienced meditators were presented with unpleasant or painful stimuli during a meditative state (Gard et al., 2012) or a baseline state (Grant, Courtemanche, & Rainville, 2011), sensory processing regions of the brain showed greater activation, and prefrontal regions appeared to decrease in activation, representing a lack of effortful regulation (e.g. reappraisal). When beginning mindfulness practice, before an automatic accepting stance develops, mindfulness might first intervene in the response modulation stage. For example, after an emotional response has occurred, beginners in mindfulness may first attempt to reduce their reactivity by focusing on their present-moment experience as it unfolds (thoughts, feelings, sensations, breath), and then reappraise the situation. With additional practice, mindfulness may be available earlier to influence attentional deployment, as one can automatically deploy 'mindful attention', effortlessly bringing a non-judgemental and accepting awareness to an emotionally charged situation, and moving through the emotion regulation stages with less reactivity and greater regulatory flexibility. Future research is needed to investigate the relationship between levels of expertise in mindfulness and the temporal process of emotion regulation.

Conclusion

Over the last two decades, there has been a great deal of wonderful theoretical and empirical development of mindfulness and emotion regulation processes in the social psychology literature. Yet, the growth of these two literatures has occurred in parallel, with little integration. Our hope has been to highlight potential points of synthesis, with an eye towards considering how mindfulness might impact emotion regulation processes, and in turn how these emotion regulation dynamics might help explain a broad range of outcomes.

References

Aldao, A., & Nolen-Hoeksema, S. (2010). Specificity of cognitive emotion regulation strategies: A transdiagnostic examination. *Behaviour Research and Therapy, 48*(10), 974–983.

Andersen, S. L., & Teicher, M. H. (2008). Stress, sensitive periods and maturational events in adolescent depression. *Trends in Neurosciences, 31*(4), 183–191.

Arch, J. J., & Craske, M. G. (2010). Laboratory stressors in clinically anxious and non-anxious individuals: The moderating role of mindfulness. *Behaviour Research and Therapy, 48*(6), 495–505.

Aspinwall, L. G., & Taylor, S. E. (1997). A stitch in time: Self-regulation and proactive coping. *Psychological Bulletin, 121*(3), 417–436.

Baer, R. A. (2003). Mindfulness training as a clinical intervention: A conceptual and empirical review. *Clinical Psychology: Science and Practice, 10*(2), 125–143.

Barnes, S., Brown, K. W., Krusemark, E., Campbell, W. K., & Rogge, R. D. (2007). The role of mindfulness in romantic relationship satisfaction and responses to relationship stress. *Journal of Marital and Family Therapy, 33*(4), 482–500.

Baumeister, R. F., & Leary, M. R. (1995). The need to belong: Desire for interpersonal attachments as a fundamental human motivation. *Psychological Bulletin, 117*(3), 497–529.

Baumeister, R. F., & Tice, D. M. (1990). Point-counterpoints: Anxiety and social exclusion. *Journal of Social and Clinical Psychology, 9*(2), 165.

Bonanno, G. A., & Burton, C. L. (2013). Regulatory flexibility: An individual differences perspective on coping and emotion regulation. *Perspectives on Psychological Science, 8*(6), 591–612.

Britton, W. B., Shahar, B., Szepsenwol, O., & Jacobs, W. J. (2012). Mindfulness-based cognitive therapy improves emotional reactivity to social stress: Results from a randomized controlled trial. *Behavior Therapy, 43*(2), 365–380.

Brodetrick, P. C. (2005). Mindfulness and coping with dysphoric mood: Contrasts with rumination and distraction. *Cognitive Therapy and Research, 29*(5), 501–510.

Brown, K. W., Goodman, R. J., & Inzlicht, M. (2013). Dispositional mindfulness and the attenuation of neural responses to emotional stimuli. *Social Cognitive and Affective Neuroscience, 8*(1), 93–99.

Brown, K. W., & Ryan, R. M. (2003). The benefits of being present: Mindfulness and its role in psychological well-being. *Journal of Personality and Social Psychology, 84*(4), 822–848.

Brown, K. W., Ryan, R. M., & Creswell, J. D. (2007). Mindfulness: Theoretical foundations and evidence for its salutary effects. *Psychological Inquiry, 18*(4), 211–237.

Brown, K. W., Weinstein, N., & Creswell, J. D. (2012). Trait mindfulness modulates neuroendocrine and affective responses to social evaluative threat. *Psychoneuroendocrinology, 37*(12), 2037–2041.

Carson, J. W., Carson, K. M., Gil, K. M., & Baucom, D. H. (2004). Mindfulness-based relationship enhancement. *Behavior Therapy, 35*(3), 471–494.

Carver, C. S., Scheier, M. F., & Weintraub, J. K. (1989). Assessing coping strategies: A theoretically based approach. *Journal of Personality and Social Psychology, 56*(2), 267–283.

Chambers, R., Gullone, E., & Allen, N. B. (2009). Mindful emotion regulation: An integrative review. *Clinical Psychology Review, 29*(6), 560–572.

Creswell, J. D., Irwin, M. R., Burklund, L. J., Lieberman, M. D., Arevalo, J. M. G., Ma, J., & Cole, S. W. (2012). Mindfulness-based stress reduction training reduces loneliness and pro-inflammatory gene expression in older adults: A small randomized controlled trial. *Brain, Behavior, and Immunity, 26*(7), 1095–1101.

Creswell, J. D., & Lindsay, E. K. (2014). How does mindfulness training affect health? A mindfulness stress buffering account. *Current Directions in Psychological Science, 23*(6), 401–407.

Creswell, J. D., Pacilio, L. E., Lindsay, E. K., & Brown, K. W. (2014). Brief mindfulness meditation training alters psychological and neuroendocrine responses to social evaluative stress. *Psychoneuroendocrinology, 44*, 1–12.

Creswell, J. D., Way, B. M., Eisenberger, N. I., & Lieberman, M. D. (2007). Neural correlates of dispositional mindfulness during affect labeling. *Psychosomatic Medicine, 69*(6), 560–565.

Desrosiers, A., Vine, V., Klemanski, D. H., & Nolen-Hoeksema, S. (2013). Mindfulness and emotion regulation in depression and anxiety: Common and distinct mechanisms of action. *Depression and Anxiety, 30*(7), 654–661.

Farb, N. A. S., Segal, Z. V., Mayberg, H., Bean, J., McKeon, D., Fatima, Z., & Anderson, A. K. (2007). Attending to the present: Mindfulness meditation reveals distinct neural modes of self-reference. *Social Cognitive and Affective Neuroscience, 2*(4), 313–322.

Feldman, G., Greeson, J., & Senville, J. (2010). Differential effects of mindful breathing, progressive muscle relaxation, and loving-kindness meditation on decentering and negative reactions to repetitive thoughts. *Behaviour Research and Therapy, 48*(10), 1002–1011.

Fresco, D. M., Moore, M. T., van Dulmen, M. H. M., Segal, Z. V., Ma, S. H., Teasdale, J. D., & Williams, J. M. G. (2007). Initial Psychometric Properties of the Experiences Questionnaire: Validation of a self-report measure of decentering. *Behavior Therapy, 38*(3), 234–246.

Gard, T., Hölzel, B. K., Sack, A. T., Hempel, H., Lazar, S. W., Vaitl, D., & Ott, U. (2012). Pain attenuation through mindfulness is associated with decreased cognitive control and increased sensory processing in the Brain. *Cerebral Cortex, 22*(11), 2692–2702.

Garland, E., Gaylord, S., & Park, J. (2009). The role of mindfulness in positive reappraisal. *EXPLORE: The Journal of Science and Healing, 5*(1), 37–44.

Goldin, P. R., & Gross, J. J. (2010). Effects of mindfulness-based stress reduction (MBSR) on emotion regulation in social anxiety disorder. *Emotion, 10*(1), 83–91.

Grant, J. A., Courtemanche, J., & Rainville, P. (2011). A non-elaborative mental stance and decoupling of executive and pain-related cortices predicts low pain sensitivity in Zen meditators. *PAIN, 152*(1), 150–156.

Gross, J. J. (1998). Antecedent- and response-focused emotion regulation: Divergent consequences for experience, expression, and physiology. *Journal of Personality and Social Psychology, 74*(1), 224–237.

Gross, J. J. (2002). Emotion regulation: Affective, cognitive, and social consequences. *Psychophysiology, 39*(3), 281–291.

Gross, J. J. (2015). Emotion regulation: Current status and future prospects. *Psychological Inquiry, 26*(1), 1–26.

Hayes-Skelton, S., & Graham, J. (2013). Decentering as a common link among mindfulness, cognitive reappraisal, and social anxiety. *Behavioural and Cognitive Psychotherapy, 41*(3), 317–328.

Heppner, W. L., Spears, C. A., Vidrine, J. I., & Wetter, D. W. (2015). Mindfulness and emotion regulation. In B. D. Ostafin, M. D. Robinson, & B. P. Meier (Eds.), *Handbook of mindfulness and self-regulation* (pp. 107–120). New York: Springer.

Hoge, E. A., Bui, E., Marques, L., Metcalf, C. A., Morris, L. K., Robinaugh, D. J., Simon, N. M. (2013). Randomized controlled trial of mindfulness meditation for generalized anxiety disorder: Effects on anxiety and stress reactivity. *The Journal of Clinical Psychiatry, 74*(8), 786–792.

Hölzel, B. K., Hoge, E. A., Greve, D. N., Gard, T., Creswell, J. D., Brown, K. W., & Lazar, S. W. (2013). Neural mechanisms of symptom improvements in generalized anxiety disorder following mindfulness training. *NeuroImage: Clinical, 2*, 448–458.

Hölzel, B. K., Lazar, S. W., Gard, T., Schuman-Olivier, Z., Vago, D. R., & Ott, U. (2011). How does mindfulness meditation work? Proposing mechanisms of action from a conceptual and neural perspective. *Perspectives on Psychological Science, 6*(6), 537–559.

Jazaieri, H., Morrison, A. S., Goldin, P. R., & Gross, J. J. (2015). The role of emotion and emotion regulation in social anxiety disorder. *Current Psychiatry Reports, 17*, 1–9.

Jha, A. P., Krompinger, J., & Baime, M. J. (2007). Mindfulness training modifies subsystems of attention. *Cognitive, Affective, & Behavioral Neuroscience, 7*(2), 109–119.

Kabat-Zinn, J., & Hanh, T. N. (2009). *Full catastrophe living: Using the wisdom of your body and mind to face stress, pain, and illness.* New York: Random House Publishing Group.

Karremans, J. C., Schellekens, M. P. J., & Kappen, G. (2015). Bridging the sciences of mindfulness and romantic relationships: A theoretical model and research agenda. *Personality and Social Psychology Review, 21*, 29–49.

Kuyken, W., Byford, S., Taylor, R. S., Watkins, E., Holden, E., White, K., Teasdale, J. D. (2008). Mindfulness-based cognitive therapy to prevent relapse in recurrent depression. *Journal of Consulting and Clinical Psychology, 76*(6), 966–978.

Lebois, L. A. M., Papies, E. K., Gopinath, K., Cabanban, R., Quigley, K. S., Krishnamurthy, V., . . . Barsalou, L. W. (2015). A shift in perspective: Decentering through mindful attention to imagined stressful events. *Neuropsychologia, 75*, 505–524.

Lindsay, E. K., & Creswell, J. D. (2017). Mechanisms of mindfulness training: Monitor and acceptance theory. *Clinical Psychology Review, 51*, 48–59.

Modinos, G., Ormel, J., & Aleman, A. (2010). Individual differences in dispositional mindfulness and brain activity involved in reappraisal of emotion. *Social Cognitive and Affective Neuroscience, 5*(4), 369–377.

Molet, M., Macquet, B., Lefebvre, O., & Williams, K. D. (2013). A focused attention intervention for coping with ostracism. *Consciousness and Cognition, 22*(4), 1262–1270.

Nyklíček, I., Dijksman, S. C., Lenders, P. J., Fonteijn, W. A., & Koolen, J. J. (2014). A brief mindfulness based intervention for increase in emotional well-being and quality of life in Percutaneous Coronary Intervention (PCI) patients: The MindfulHeart randomized controlled trial. *Journal of Behavioral Medicine, 37*(1), 135–144.

Quaglia, J. T., Brown, K. W., Lindsay, E. K., Creswell, J. D., & Goodman, R. J. (2014). From conceptualization to operationalization of mindfulness. *Handbook of mindfulness: Theory, research, and practice* (pp. 151–170). New York: Guilford Press.

Rasmussen, M. K., & Pidgeon, A. M. (2010). The direct and indirect benefits of dispositional mindfulness on self-esteem and social anxiety. *Anxiety, Stress and Coping, 24*(2), 227–233.

Shikatani, B., Antony, M. M., Kuo, J. R., & Cassin, S. E. (2014). The impact of cognitive restructuring and mindfulness strategies on postevent processing and affect in social anxiety disorder. *Journal of Anxiety Disorders, 28*(6), 570–579.

Tang, Y-Y., Ma, Y., Wang, J., Fan, Y., Feng, S., & Lu, Q. (2007). Short-term meditation training improves attention and self-regulation. *Proceedings of the National Academy of Sciences, 104*(43), 17152–17156.

Teper, R., & Inzlicht, M. (2013). Meditation, mindfulness and executive control: The importance of emotional acceptance and brain-based performance monitoring. *Social Cognitive and Affective Neuroscience, 8*(1), 85–92.

Vago, D. R., & Nakamura, Y. (2011). Selective attentional bias towards pain-related threat in fibromyalgia: Preliminary evidence for effects of mindfulness meditation training. *Cognitive Therapy and Research, 35*(6), 581–594.

Webb, T. L., Miles, E., & Sheeran, P. (2012). Dealing with feeling: A meta-analysis of the effectiveness of strategies derived from the process model of emotion regulation. *Psychological Bulletin, 138*(4), 775–808.

Weinstein, N., Brown, K. W., & Ryan, R. M. (2009). A multi-method examination of the effects of mindfulness on stress attribution, coping, and emotional well-being. *Journal of Research in Personality, 43*(3), 374–385.

7

MINDFULNESS AND HEALTH BEHAVIOUR

Examining the roles of attention regulation and decentering

Esther K. Papies

Since the introduction of mindfulness-based stress reduction by Kabat-Zinn (1982), mindfulness-based interventions have been shown to be effective for dealing with a variety of conditions like stress and anxiety, and to generally improve psychological well-being (for reviews, see Baer, 2003; Goyal, Singh, Sibinga et al., 2014; Grossman, Niemann, Schmidt, & Walach, 2004). More recently, mindfulness has also gained increasing interest with regard to health behaviours, for example, eating, smoking, and alcohol use. Similarly, mindfulness has become increasingly popular as a tool for initiating behaviour change, both by lay individuals who study mindfulness from self-help books or courses, and by scientists who investigate the effects of mindfulness-based interventions systematically. While this work has suggested that mindfulness is a powerful approach to stimulate healthy behaviour, we only have limited insights into the psychological mechanisms underlying these effects. Therefore, the current chapter presents a review of recent work on mindfulness and health behaviour, particularly with a view to elucidating its underlying mechanisms. This may contribute to both further systematic research as well as targeted applications of mindfulness to facilitate health behaviour change.

For the sake of the current analysis and based on existing conceptualizations (Bishop et al., 2004; Lutz, Jha, Dunne, & Saron, 2015), mindfulness will be regarded as a state that is characterized by two components, namely (1) the regulation of attention, and (2) meta-cognitive awareness and insight into the nature of one's experiences, which allows one to view them in a non-judgemental manner as "passing events in the mind" (Bishop et al., 2004, p. 234). Attention regulation refers to the ability to monitor, control, and sustain attention, including maintaining it for an extended period of time on a chosen object. This part of mindfulness is trained in various types of meditation (Lutz, Slagter, Dunne, & Davidson, 2008), also referred to as *śamatha* or concentration practice (Grabovac, Lau, & Willett, 2011). Typically, meditation in mindfulness training instructs participants to direct their attention to whatever they are experiencing in the present moment, which over time increases one's present-moment awareness (Bishop et al., 2004; Brown & Ryan, 2003).

The second mindfulness component will be referred to as "decentering" here, but it strongly resembles what has been described as "re-perceiving", cognitive insight, or "cognitive defusion" (Chambers, Gullone, & Allen, 2009; Grabovac et al., 2011; Hayes & Wilson, 2003; Shapiro, Carlson, Astin, & Freedman, 2006). While people typically get deeply immersed in their thoughts and experience them as very compelling and real, decentering reflects the meta-cognitive awareness that one's thoughts and experiences are in essence no more than mental events. In other words, decentering refers to the insight that even the most compelling simulations, intense emotions, and realistic thoughts occur only in one's mind, where one can observe them arise and dissipate without having to act on them in any way (see Papies, Pronk, Keesman, & Barsalou, 2015). Typically, mindfulness training teaches participants this perspective with regard to emotional and physical states they may experience during meditation practice and in daily life, which facilitates acceptance and non-reactivity to both pleasant and unpleasant experiences (Grabovac et al., 2011).

In this chapter I will first briefly review how comprehensive mindfulness interventions, as well as self-reported mindfulness skills reflecting both of these components, have been shown to affect health behaviour. Then I will lay out critical processes in the regulation of health behaviour, and next I will discuss studies investigating effects of attention processes and decentering on these processes separately. Finally, I will turn to the ways that attention regulation and decentering interact and complement each other, discuss the possibility of the domain-specificity of mindfulness effects, and end the chapter with some broader conclusions.

Effects of comprehensive mindfulness interventions and skills on health behaviour

A significant number of studies to date have shown effects of comprehensive mindfulness interventions and of mindfulness-related skills on health behaviour. Let us first briefly discuss findings in the domain of eating and weight control, and then turn to research on smoking and alcohol use. It should be noted that the literature review in this chapter is not designed to be exhaustive, but rather to illustrate the developments in the field and the potential mechanisms underlying mindfulness effects. In addition, the domains of eating behaviour, smoking, and alcohol use simply serve to illustrate basic processes that are most likely applicable to other health behaviours as well.

Eating behaviour

A number of studies have shown that mindfulness interventions can lead to healthier eating patterns among both healthy and eating-disordered participants. In one experiment among healthy participants, for example, a brief laboratory training that focused on both awareness during eating and on developing a non-judgemental attitude, led to a reduction in impulsive choices in a delay-discounting task, compared to a nutrition information control condition (Hendrickson & Rasmussen, 2013). Similarly, brief body scan exercises combining attention regulation with a non-judgemental attitude have been shown to prevent overeating on attractive but unhealthy foods in a laboratory context (Jordan, Wang, Donatoni, & Meier, 2014; Marchiori & Papies, 2014). In line with these experimental findings, correlational studies have shown that individual differences in skills that reflect mindfulness, such as eating and responding to food cues with awareness, are associated with reduced intake of unhealthy foods and lower body mass index (Beshara, Hutchinson, & Wilson, 2013; Framson et al., 2009; Jordan et al., 2014). Together, these findings suggest that mindfulness skills can reduce the appeal of unhealthy food temptations among healthy individuals.

Among participants with disordered eating, Alberts and colleagues have shown that in comparison to a wait-list control group, participants who received a mindfulness-based intervention displayed reduced food cravings and problematic food-related thinking after an 8-week period (Alberts, Thewissen, & Raes, 2012). The mindfulness intervention contained both an attention regulation component – such as increasing awareness of thoughts, physical states, and eating-related sensations – and an attitudinal component promoting a non-judging approach to one's experiences. Focusing specifically on patients with binge-eating disorder, Kristeller and colleagues showed similar mindfulness-based interventions to reduce binge eating and associated pathology (Kristeller & Hallett, 1999; Kristeller, Wolever, & Sheets, 2014; see Wanden-Berghe, Sanz-Valero, & Wanden-Berghe, 2010, for a review of further, small-scale studies). Synthesizing these literatures, O'Reilly and colleagues (2014) and Katterman and colleagues (2014) reviewed about 20 studies that included mindfulness components targeted at eating behaviour, and found that the majority reported improvements in disordered eating, and to a lesser degree, reductions in body weight.

Smoking and alcohol use

Fewer but similar findings have been reported in the areas of smoking and alcohol use (see also Chiesa & Serretti, 2014, for a systematic review across substance abuse disorders). Brewer and colleagues (2011), for example, showed that a mindfulness intervention containing both attention and decentering elements (e.g. awareness of craving cues, adopting a non-judgemental perspective) reduced cigarette consumption among smokers motivated to quit more than among participants in a control intervention. Bowen and Marlatt (2009) showed that applying mindfulness principles to dealing with cue-elicited cravings reduced smoking over a 7-day follow-up period, and it weakened the association between smoking urges and actual smoking. Elwafi et al. (2013) further showed that this craving-smoking link reduction was stronger for participants who applied mindfulness principles more in their daily lives during the 4 weeks of treatment. In a more recent study, Ruscio and colleagues showed that a brief, 3-session mindfulness intervention, again providing instructions for attention regulation as well as for decentering, reduced negative affect, cravings, and number of cigarettes smoked over a 2-week period, compared to an active control condition (Ruscio, Muench, Brede, & Waters, 2015). In the domain of alcohol use, Brewer et al. (2009) and Garland et al. (2010) found reduced reactivity to typical triggers of alcohol use, such as descriptions of stressful events and pictures of alcohol, among participants who had completed a mindfulness intervention, and a negative association of trait mindfulness with attentional bias for alcohol cues (Garland, Boettiger, Gaylord, Chanon, & Howard, 2012). Extending this to behavioural effects, a large randomized clinical trial showed that mindfulness-based relapse prevention reduced substance use and heavy drinking at 12-month follow-up, compared to control treatments (Bowen et al., 2014).

Levin, Luoma, & Haeger (2015) recently reviewed work showing a decoupling between typical triggers of smoking and alcohol use, such as negative affect and cravings, and actual use of these substances. They identified a small number of studies in which a mindfulness-based intervention or trait mindfulness skills modulated the link between such triggers and substance use, suggesting that mindfulness can indeed change the effects of one's internal experiences, such as cravings, on behaviour.

Although the effect of mindfulness in these studies is sometimes weak and limited by methodological concerns (see Chiesa & Serretti, 2014), these studies on comprehensive mindfulness interventions suggest that mindfulness can have beneficial effects on health behaviour, for example, by reducing problematic eating behaviour and decreasing the effects of cravings on cigarettes and alcohol use. How do mindfulness interventions work to achieve these effects?

Potential roles for attention regulation and decentering in health behaviour

To understand the mechanisms by which mindfulness could affect health behaviour, let us first consider some critical processes in the regulation of health behaviour, and then discuss how the mindfulness components of attention regulation and decentering could affect them (for similar analyses of how comprehensive mindfulness interventions can target addictive behaviours, see for example Brewer, Elwafi, & Davis, 2012; Witkiewitz, Marlatt, & Walker, 2005).

Recent research shows how people often automatically act on short-term rewards, despite the best long-term intentions (e.g. Hofmann, Friese, & Wiers, 2008; Webb & Sheeran, 2006). Impulsive and also addictive behaviours to obtain short-term rewards are typically triggered by an environmental cue, for example, the smell of tasty food, or by an internal state, such as feeling stressed. Often, such cues go unnoticed, and the processes by which they affect health behaviour are automatic in the sense of being unintentional and occurring outside of conscious awareness (e.g. Barsalou, Chapter 3 in this volume; Papies, 2016; Papies & Barsalou, 2015). As a result, for example, seeing tasty food in a deli window can trigger buying and eating a rich piece of cake, despite one's dieting intentions and in the absence of hunger.

Successful health behaviour therefore relies on effective monitoring of internal and external cues, making it more likely that a person will become aware of the cues and processes affecting their behaviour, so that more deliberate courses of action become possible (see also Elkins-Brown, Teper, & Inzlicht, Chapter 5 in this volume). With effective monitoring, one can detect when a tempting situation arises and can prepare appropriate action, for example, walking away from a drinking contest at a party, in order to prevent binge drinking (see Hagger et al., 2011). Similarly, monitoring can entail assessing one's behaviour in relation to one's standards, for example, comparing one's food intake to one's eating goals, in order to prevent mindless overeating on tasty food (see Versluis & Papies, 2016; Ward & Mann, 2000).

In many cases, however, internal or external cues trigger a desire or conscious craving for a certain substance that is hard to simply walk away from, especially in case of an addiction (for a review, see for example Kavanagh, Andrade, & May, 2005; Witkiewitz et al., 2005). Desire and cravings have been described as the motivation and strong urge, respectively, to consume a certain substance, arising from expectations of reward based on earlier consumptive experiences (e.g. Brewer et al., 2012; Kavanagh et al., 2005; Papies & Barsalou, 2015). Once representations of rewarding consumption experiences have been established, the mere exposure to a cue associated with enjoying temping food, smoking, or drinking alcohol, can be enough to trigger a vivid and seemingly "real" simulation of consuming and enjoying the substance, leading to the experience of desire and possibly, to actual consumption behaviour (Papies & Barsalou, 2015). Crucially, applying a decentered perspective to these simulations can make them less subjectively real and compelling, or in Buddhist terms, "empty". In other words, realizing that these simulations, as vivid and rewarding as they may seem, are merely mental events that will dissipate naturally, can reduce their motivational power.

When cravings do arise, healthy choices may still result from trying to counter them with thoughts of the conflicting goal (Papies, Stroebe, & Aarts, 2008), or again, from applying a decentered perspective to one's desire thoughts by realizing their nature as mere mental events that will dissipate naturally. Executive attention, or the ability to control one's attention, may then again be important to maintain the decentered perspective as well as information about the desired behaviour in working memory, and to shield it from interference from undesired response tendencies (Engle, 2002; Hofmann, Gschwendner, Friese, Wiers, & Schmitt, 2008).

As this brief analysis has shown, the mindfulness components of attention regulation and decentering could affect the processes that regulate health behaviour at various points. Attentional processes can support the detection of tempting cues, the monitoring of one's behaviour, and the activation and maintenance of one's long-term goals. Decentering can prevent the development of desire from reward cues at various points, as one sees that one's rewarding simulations of consuming the substance are mere mental events. Further, decentering can help to reduce desire and prevent its effects on behaviour in those cases where it did develop, thus decoupling the link between desire and behaviour as was described above.

Importantly, the present analysis suggests specific effects of these mindfulness components on processes that underlie health behaviour. So far, however, no research has tested this account directly and comprehensively. The studies described in the first part of this chapter contained elements that most likely affected both mindfulness components, so that their respective contributions to the effects on health behaviours cannot be inferred. The work described in the next sections speaks more directly to the effects of attention regulation and decentering on health behaviour, even if not all of it was designed to specifically examine mindfulness effects.

Attention regulation and decentering as mindfulness mechanisms

For both attentional processes and decentering, let us now look at how each of these components is affected by mindfulness training, then how they affect health behaviour, and finally, how these mechanisms could be underlying the mindfulness effects on health behaviour that are reported in the literature.

Attention regulation

A large number of studies have shown that mindfulness training influences attentional processes. To name a few examples, mindfulness meditation has been found to improve the orienting of attention (Jha, Krompinger, & Baime, 2007), the processing of interoceptive signals (Farb, Segal, & Anderson, 2013), attentional control (e.g. Chambers, Lo, & Allen, 2008; Moore, Gruber, Derose, & Malinowski, 2012), and sustained attention (Zeidan, Johnson, Diamond, David, & Goolkasian, 2010). Recent reviews and a meta-analysis have confirmed such findings across studies and shown that mindfulness meditation improves core attentional processes (Chiesa, Calati, & Serretti, 2011; Sedlmeier et al., 2012). These processes parallel those that are trained during a session of concentrative meditation practice where one directs attention to a chosen object, maintains attention, and responds to mind-wandering by bringing attention back to the chosen object (see Hasenkamp, Wilson-Mendenhall, Duncan, & Barsalou, 2012).

Research has also shown that these attentional processes affect health behaviour in critical ways. Individuals with better executive attention, for example, are better able to override their impulses and act in line with long-term goals, such as dieting (Hofmann, Gschwendner et al., 2008), as are individuals who have completed a mindfulness training (Ostafin, Bauer, & Myxter, 2012). Reduced attention during eating decreases taste sensitivity (van der Wal & van Dillen, 2013) and increases unhealthy intake (Ward & Mann, 2000). In contrast, directing attention toward one's eating can prevent later overeating (Higgs & Donohoe, 2011), and training to systematically direct attention away from tempting food cues can reduce cravings and consumption (Kemps, Tiggemann, Orr, & Grear, 2014). Training attention away from tempting cues seems less effective in the domains of alcohol and smoking, but findings do suggest that repeatedly directing attention *toward* alcohol and tobacco cues can *increase* craving and consumption among heavy users (Field & Eastwood, 2005; Schoenmakers et al., 2010). Selective attention toward substance-related cues has been found to be a predictor of craving more generally (Franken, 2003), again pointing to the central role of attentional processes.

In line with the analysis of health behaviour presented earlier, these findings indicate that the way an individual directs and regulates attention in a tempting environment can be of critical importance for health behaviour. Thus, mindfulness may be effective because the attention regulation component of mindfulness increases one's ability to accurately detect internal and external cues that trigger craving, to direct attention away from desire-inducing and toward desire-reducing information, and to keep one's long-term goals in mind. Although awaiting direct empirical testing, this account may explain how mindfulness interventions affect health behaviour through improved attention regulation skills.

Decentering

Less research has focused specifically on the decentering component of mindfulness. However, a number of studies show that mindfulness is associated with increased decentering as assessed by self-report measures (Davis, Lau, & Cairns, 2009; Hayes-Skelton & Graham, 2013; Lau et al., 2006), and that completing a mindfulness training increases decentering abilities (Hoge et al., 2014; Lau et al., 2006). Whereas no clear behavioural or neural markers of decentering currently exist, research further suggests that mindfulness training alters the processing of emotional stimuli in ways that are consistent with less intense and reactive processing, in line with a decentered perspective (Desbordes et al., 2012; Hölzel et al., 2013; Lebois et al., 2015; Ostafin, Brooks, & Laitem, 2014). These processes again parallel those that are trained during mindfulness practice and in various schools of meditation, as one practices the capacity to break the "time traveling" and subjective realism that typically characterize our mental experiences (Dunne, 2011; Papies, Barsalou, & Custers, 2012).

Importantly, a number of experimental studies have recently demonstrated the effects of decentering on health-related cognition and behaviour. In the domain of eating behaviour, Papies and colleagues (2012, 2015) have shown that teaching non-meditators to apply a decentered perspective by observing their responses to food pictures as mere mental events can reduce approach impulses toward tempting food as well as actual unhealthy choices and eating behaviour, especially among hungry participants. In other words, once participants realized that the eating and enjoyment thoughts that the food pictures typically trigger are merely mental events, the desire for these foods was strongly reduced, and resisting them became easier. Jenkins and Tapper (2014) showed that applying such a decentering perspective to chocolate helped participants reduce chocolate intake over a 5-day period, and Lacaille and colleagues (2014) demonstrated that training decentering was more effective than other mindfulness-based skills in preventing and reducing chocolate craving. Similar approaches, based on the so-called urge-surfing technique where one learns to accept one's cravings and let them naturally dissipate, have been shown to be beneficial in the domain of smoking (Rogojanski, Vettese, & Antony, 2011). Finally, correlational studies suggest that decentering skills are related to reduced food cravings in experienced meditators (Keesman, Aarts, Häfner, & Papies, 2016; Papies, van Winckel, & Keesman, 2016).

Again in line with the analysis of health behaviour presented earlier, these findings indicate that the ability to apply a decentered perspective to tempting stimuli can be of critical importance for health behaviour. Mindfulness training may be effective as the decentering component increases one's ability to view the reward-related thoughts that typically lead to full-blown cravings as mere mental events. Realizing that the reward anticipated from consumption is merely a passing mental state makes a tempting stimulus much less inherently attractive, and can prevent impulses and cravings. As a result, deliberate processes supporting one's long-term goals are more likely to affect behaviour. In addition, applying decentering repeatedly may lead to a lasting change in the representation of tempting stimuli, so that they will be less likely to activate rewarding consumption simulations later (Barsalou, Chapter 3 in this volume; Papies et al., 2015). Although again awaiting direct empirical testing, this account may explain how mindfulness interventions affect health behaviour through decentering skills.

Interactions of attention regulation and decentering

So far, we have looked mainly at the separate roles of attention regulation and decentering skills in health behaviour. In actual mindfulness training, however, these two skills complement and support each other and are typically trained together, and it seems likely that such interactions also occur in health behaviour (Papies et al., 2015). As suggested in Papies et al. (2015), training attention regulation will be much easier if combined with the insight of decentring. During meditation practice, distractions will inevitably arise, for example, while one is focusing attention on one's breath. Applying decentring will allow one to perceive such distractions as mere mental events, making it less likely to get caught up in them and thus easier to return to one's chosen object of attention. This way, decentering can facilitate the training of attention regulation during meditation practice, or "on the cushion". In a similar manner, decentring can support the application of attention regulation skills in one's daily life, or "off the cushion". As an example, consider a dinner party with good conversation and attractive food. Here, keeping one's overall health goals in mind so that one can consistently pursue them will be easier if one applies decentering and thus perceives food temptations that would otherwise lead to unhealthy behaviours as less inherently attractive.

Conversely, it can be argued that good skills in attention regulation support both the training of and the real-life application of decentering. While research has shown that decentering can be learned and applied by non-meditators after a very brief training (e.g. Jenkins & Tapper, 2014; Papies et al., 2012, 2015), the application of this perspective over an extended period of time will benefit from good skills in attention regulation. In particular, maintaining a decentered perspective during one's meditation means that a particular processing mode has to be kept active in working memory in order to apply it directly to distractions as they arise, before one gets carried off in associative thought. Similarly, applying decentering in real-world situations without being prompted to do so by an experimenter or mindfulness trainer and while being exposed to various distractions is much easier if supported by good attentional skills. These will facilitate both the detection of critical opportunities to apply decentering, as well as the return to a decentered perspective after possible interruptions (see also Hasenkamp et al., 2012).

As this brief discussion illustrates, attention regulation and decentering seem to play unique roles in the effects of mindfulness interventions on health behaviour, but they also support and complement each other. Thus, while an analysis of these separate components is useful for understanding the mechanisms of mindfulness, and targeted applications of these components may be useful for particular issues (see Papies et al., 2015), mindfulness may in most cases be applied most effectively if both decentering and attention regulation skills are trained.

Domain-specificity of mindfulness effects

Most of the mindfulness interventions described here were targeted toward a specific behaviour and delivered with a particular long-term goal in mind, for example, to reduce alcohol consumption or food cravings. While these domain-specific interventions have demonstrated promising effects, a critical look at the literature suggests that general mindfulness programs (e.g. mindfulness-based stress reduction, or MBSR), have only limited effects on specific health behaviours. Indeed, a recent meta-analysis found evidence for effectiveness of these programs for dealing with depression, pain, and anxiety, but no effects on specific outcomes that were not targeted directly by the programs, like healthy eating behaviours and body weight (Goyal et al., 2014). Thus, mindfulness interventions for health behaviour may be most effective if they are targeted at a specific domain.

One possible reason for this mindfulness specificity may be a person's motivation to change (see also Karremans & Kappen, Chapter 8 in this volume). A participant in a stress-reduction program, for example, may not be particularly motivated to reduce smoking and lose weight, in addition to dealing with stress, so that changes on such specific behaviours are less likely to occur. Alternatively, participants may not realize that the skills they learn – for example, for dealing with stress and negative affect – can also help them deal with reward-related issues, like cravings and desires.

Finally, the mechanisms potentially underlying the mindfulness effects as discussed earlier may also help us understand why mindfulness works best if it is delivered in a domain-specific way. A specific mindfulness training is more likely to include practices that train participants in becoming aware of the relevant internal and external cues affecting their behaviour, for example, the cues that trigger cigarette craving, or that precipitate overeating. Similarly, a domain-specific training is more likely to be effective for developing decentering skills for exactly those cravings that challenge participants most, for example, by having participants apply it directly to the thoughts and sensations associated with cigarette cravings (see, for example, the application of the urge-surfing technique in Bowen & Marlatt, 2009). In other words, both attention regulation and decentering may be most effective if they are situated (see Papies, 2016), such that they are trained in a domain that is relevant to participants, and if the content that these skills are trained on is critical to the problems that participants experience.

It should be noted that a few studies have shown associations between general mindfulness skills and specific health behaviours or their predictors. A brief, general mindfulness training, for example, reduced the effect of automatic processes on alcohol thoughts and drinking behaviour (Ostafin et al., 2012) and lead to healthier eating (Jordan et al., 2014); and self-reported general mindfulness was associated with stronger enactment of one's physical activity intentions (Chatzisarantis & Hagger, 2007), and with a reduced tendency to eat in response to stress and strong emotions (Pidgeon, Lacota, & Champion, 2012). The findings on the domain specificity of mindfulness, however, suggest that such effects might be stronger if mindfulness skills were trained or assessed specifically with regard to the critical health behaviours under study.

Summary and conclusions

In this chapter, I have examined how mindfulness interventions may affect health behaviour through affecting attention regulation and decentering. By analyzing the processes that underlie the regulation of health behaviour, such as the detection of tempting cues, the maintenance of health goals in working memory, and the prevention and regulation of craving, we have seen that mindfulness effects can be understood as effects of either attention regulation, or the application of a decentered perspective to temptations. Although various lines of research support this account in indirect ways, future research should examine these mechanisms directly, so that a more detailed understanding of mindfulness mechanisms can further support their most effective application.

Acknowledgement

I am grateful to Johan Karremans and Lawrence W. Barsalou for helpful comments on an earlier version of this chapter.

References

Alberts, H. J. E. M., Thewissen, R., & Raes, L. (2012). Dealing with problematic eating behaviour. The effects of a mindfulness-based intervention on eating behaviour, food cravings, dichotomous thinking and body image concern. *Appetite, 58*(3), 847–851.

Baer, R. A. (2003). Mindfulness training as a clinical intervention: A conceptual and empirical review. *Clinical Psychology: Science and Practice, 10*(2), 125–143.

Beshara, M., Hutchinson, A. D., & Wilson, C. (2013). Does mindfulness matter? Everyday mindfulness, mindful eating and self-reported serving size of energy dense foods among a sample of South Australian adults. *Appetite, 67*, 25–29.

Bishop, S. R., Lau, M., Shapiro, S., Carlson, L., Anderson, N. D., Carmody, J., . . . Devins. (2004). Mindfulness: A proposed operational definition. *Clinical Psychology: Science and Practice, 11*(3), 230–241.

Bowen, S., & Marlatt, A. (2009, December). Surfing the urge: Brief mindfulness-based intervention for college student smokers. *Psychology of Addictive Behaviors, 23*(4), 666–671.

Bowen, S., Witkiewitz, K., Clifasefi, S. L., Grow, J., Chawla, N., Hsu, S. H., . . . Larimer, M. E. (2014). Relative efficacy of mindfulness-based relapse prevention, standard relapse prevention, and treatment as usual for substance use disorders: A randomized clinical trial. *JAMA Psychiatry, 71*(5), 547–556.

Brewer, J. A., Elwafi, H. M., & Davis, J. H. (2012). Craving to quit: Psychological models and neurobiological mechanisms of mindfulness training as treatment for addictions. *Psychology of Addictive Behaviors, 27*, 366-372.

Brewer, J. A., Mallik, S., Babuscio, T. A., Nich, C., Johnson, H. E., Deleone, C. M., . . . Rounsaville, B. J. (2011). Mindfulness training for smoking cessation: Results from a randomized controlled trial. *Drug and Alcohol Dependence, 119*(1–2), 72–80.

Brewer, J. A., Sinha, R., Chen, J. A., Michalsen, R. N., Babuscio, T. A., Nich, C., . . . Rounsaville, B. J. (2009). Mindfulness training and stress reactivity in substance abuse: Results from a randomized, controlled stage I pilot study. *Substance Abuse, 30*(4), 306–317.

Brown, K. W., & Ryan, R. M. (2003). The benefits of being present: Mindfulness and its role in psychological well-being. *Journal of Personality and Social Psychology, 84*(4), 822–848.

Chambers, R., Gullone, E., & Allen, N. B. (2009). Mindful emotion regulation: An integrative review. *Clinical Psychology Review, 29*(6), 560–572.

Chambers, R., Lo, B., & Allen, N. (2008). The impact of intensive mindfulness training on attentional control, cognitive style, and affect. *Cognitive Therapy and Research, 32*(3), 303–322.

Chatzisarantis, N. L. D., & Hagger, M. S. (2007). Mindfulness and the intention-behavior relationship within the theory of planned behavior. *Personality and Social Psychology Bulletin, 33*(5), 663–676.

Chiesa, A., Calati, R., & Serretti, A. (2011). Does mindfulness training improve cognitive abilities? A systematic review of neuropsychological findings. *Clinical Psychology Review, 31*(3), 449–464.

Chiesa, A., & Serretti, A. (2014). Are mindfulness-based interventions effective for substance use disorders? A systematic review of the evidence. *Substance Use & Misuse, 49*(5), 492–512.

Davis, K. M., Lau, M. A., & Cairns, D. R. (2009). Development and preliminary validation of a trait version of the Toronto Mindfulness Scale. *Journal of Cognitive Psychotherapy, 23*(3), 185–197.

Desbordes, G., Negi, L. T., Pace, T. W. W., Wallace, B. A., Raison, C. L., & Schwartz, E. L. (2012). Effects of mindful-attention and compassion meditation training on amygdala response to emotional stimuli in an ordinary, non-meditative state. *Frontiers in Human Neuroscience, 6*, 292.

Dunne, J. D. (2011). Toward an understanding of non-dual mindfulness. *Contemporary Buddhism, 12*(1), 71–88.

Elwafi, H. M., Witkiewitz, K., Mallik, S., Thornhill, T. A., IV, & Brewer, J. A. (2013). Mindfulness training for smoking cessation: Moderation of the relationship between craving and cigarette use. *Drug and Alcohol Dependence, 130*(1–3), 222–229.

Engle, R. W. (2002). Working memory capacity as executive attention. *Current Directions in Psychological Science, 11*(1), 19–23.

Farb, N. A. S., Segal, Z. V., & Anderson, A. K. (2013). Mindfulness meditation training alters cortical representations of interoceptive attention. *Social Cognitive and Affective Neuroscience, 8*(1), 15–26.

Field, M., & Eastwood, B. (2005). Experimental manipulation of attentional bias increases the motivation to drink alcohol. *Psychopharmacology, 183*(3), 350–357.

Framson, C., Kristal, A. R., Schenk, J. M., Littman, A. J., Zeliadt, S., & Benitez, D. (2009). Development and validation of the Mindful Eating Questionnaire. *Journal of the American Dietetic Association, 109*(8), 1439–1444.

Franken, I. H. A. (2003). Drug craving and addiction: Integrating psychological and neuropsychopharmacological approaches. *Progress in Neuro-Psychopharmacology and Biological Psychiatry, 27*(4), 563–579.

Garland, E. L., Boettiger, C. A., Gaylord, S., Chanon, V. W., & Howard, M. O. (2012). Mindfulness is inversely associated with alcohol attentional bias among recovering alcohol-dependent adults. *Cognitive Therapy and Research, 36*(5), 441–450.

Garland, E. L., Gaylord, S. A., Boettiger, C. A., & Howard, M. O. (2010). Mindfulness training modifies cognitive, affective, and physiological mechanisms implicated in alcohol dependence: Results of a randomized controlled pilot trial. *Journal of Psychoactive Drugs, 42*(2), 177–192.

Goyal, M., Singh, S., Sibinga, E. S., Gould, N. F., Rowland-Seymour, A., Sharma, R., . . . Haythornthwaite, J. A. (2014). Meditation programs for psychological stress and well-being: A systematic review and meta-analysis. *JAMA Internal Medicine, 174*(3), 357–368. http://doi.org/10.1001/jamainternmed.2013.13018

Grabovac, A. D., Lau, M. A., & Willett, B. R. (2011). Mechanisms of mindfulness: A Buddhist psychological model. *Mindfulness, 2*(3), 154–166.

Grossman, P., Niemann, L., Schmidt, S., & Walach, H. (2004). Mindfulness-based stress reduction and health benefits: A meta-analysis. *Journal of Psychosomatic Research, 57*(1), 35–43.

Hagger, M. S., Lonsdale, A., Koka, A., Hein, V., Pasi, H., Lintunen, T., & Chatzisarantis, N. L. D. (2011). An intervention to reduce alcohol consumption in undergraduate students using implementation intentions and mental simulations: A cross-national study. *International Journal of Behavioral Medicine, 19*(1), 82–96.

Hasenkamp, W., Wilson-Mendenhall, C. D., Duncan, E., & Barsalou, L. W. (2012). Mind wandering and attention during focused meditation: A fine-grained temporal analysis of fluctuating cognitive states. *NeuroImage, 59*(1), 750–760. http://doi.org/10.1016/j.neuroimage.2011.07.008

Hayes, S. C., & Wilson, K. G. (2003). Mindfulness: Method and process. *Clinical Psychology: Science and Practice, 10*(2), 161–165.

Hayes-Skelton, S., & Graham, J. (2013). Decentering as a common link among mindfulness, cognitive reappraisal, and social anxiety. *Behavioural and Cognitive Psychotherapy, 41*(3), 317–328.

Hendrickson, K. L., & Rasmussen, E. B. (2013). Effects of mindful eating training on delay and probability discounting for food and money in obese and healthy-weight individuals. *Behaviour Research and Therapy, 51*(7), 399–409.

Higgs, S., & Donohoe, J. E. (2011). Focusing on food during lunch enhances lunch memory and decreases later snack intake. *Appetite, 57*(1), 202–206.

Hofmann, W., Friese, M., & Wiers, R. W. (2008). Impulsive versus reflective influences on health behavior: A theoretical framework and empirical review. *Health Psychology Review*, *2*(2), 111–137.

Hofmann, W., Gschwendner, T., Friese, M., Wiers, R. W., & Schmitt, M. (2008). Working memory capacity and self-regulatory behavior: Toward an individual differences perspective on behavior determination by automatic versus controlled processes. *Journal of Personality and Social Psychology*, *95*(4), 962–977.

Hoge, E. A., Bui, E., Goetter, E., Robinaugh, D. J., Ojserkis, R. A., Fresco, D. M., & Simon, N. M. (2014). Change in decentering mediates improvement in anxiety in mindfulness-based stress reduction for generalized anxiety disorder. *Cognitive Therapy and Research*, *39*(2), 228–235.

Hölzel, B. K., Hoge, E. A., Greve, D. N., Gard, T., Creswell, J. D., Brown, K. W., . . . Lazar, S. W. (2013). Neural mechanisms of symptom improvements in generalized anxiety disorder following mindfulness training. *NeuroImage: Clinical*, *2*, 448–458.

Jenkins, K. T., & Tapper, K. (2014). Resisting chocolate temptation using a brief mindfulness strategy. *British Journal of Health Psychology*, *19*(3), 509–522.

Jha, A. P., Krompinger, J., & Baime, M. J. (2007). Mindfulness training modifies subsystems of attention. *Cognitive, Affective, & Behavioral Neuroscience*, *7*(2), 109–119.

Jordan, C. H., Wang, W., Donatoni, L., & Meier, B. P. (2014). Mindful eating: Trait and state mindfulness predict healthier eating behavior. *Personality and Individual Differences*, *68*, 107–111.

Kabat-Zinn, J. (1982). An outpatient program in behavioral medicine for chronic pain patients based on the practice of mindfulness meditation: Theoretical considerations and preliminary results. *General Hospital Psychiatry*, *4*(1), 33–47.

Katterman, S. N., Kleinman, B. M., Hood, M. M., Nackers, L. M., & Corsica, J. A. (2014). Mindfulness meditation as an intervention for binge eating, emotional eating, and weight loss: A systematic review. *Eating Behaviors*, *15*(2), 197–204.

Kavanagh, D. J., Andrade, J., & May, J. (2005). Imaginary relish and exquisite torture: The elaborated intrusion theory of desire. *Psychological Review*, *112*(2), 446–467.

Keesman, M., Aarts, H., Häfner, M., & Papies, E. K. (2016). Benefits of meditation experience on resilience and craving occur through decentering but not awareness. Under review.

Kemps, E., Tiggemann, M., Orr, J., & Grear, J. (2014). Attentional retraining can reduce chocolate consumption. *Journal of Experimental Psychology: Applied*, *20*(1), 94–102.

Kristeller, J. L., & Hallett, C. B. (1999). An exploratory study of a meditation-based intervention for binge eating disorder. *Journal of Health Psychology*, *4*(3), 357–363.

Kristeller, J. L., Wolever, R. Q., & Sheets, V. (2014). Mindfulness-Based Eating Awareness Training (MB-EAT) for binge eating: A randomized clinical trial. *Mindfulness*, *5*(3), 282–297.

Lacaille, J., Ly, J., Zacchia, N., Bourkas, S., Glaser, E., & Knäuper, B. (2014). The effects of three mindfulness skills on chocolate cravings. *Appetite*, *76*, 101–112.

Lau, M. A., Bishop, S. R., Segal, Z. V., Buis, T., Anderson, N. D., Carlson, L., . . . Devins, G. (2006). The Toronto Mindfulness Scale: Development and validation. *Journal of Clinical Psychology*, *62*(12), 1445–1467.

Lebois, L. A. M., Papies, E. K., Gopinath, K., Cabanban, R., Quigley, K. S., Krishnamurthy, V., . . . Barsalou, L. W. (2015). A shift in perspective: Decentering through mindful attention to imagined stressful events. *Neuropsychologia*, *75*, 505–524.

Levin, M. E., Luoma, J. B., & Haeger, J. A. (2015). Decoupling as a mechanism of change in mindfulness and acceptance: A literature review. *Behavior Modification*, *39*(6), 870–911.

Lutz, A., Jha, A. P., Dunne, J. D., & Saron, C. D. (2015). Investigating the phenomenological matrix of mindfulness-related practices from a neurocognitive perspective. *American Psychologist*, *70*(7), 632–658.

Lutz, A., Slagter, H. A., Dunne, J. D., & Davidson, R. J. (2008). Attention regulation and monitoring in meditation. *Trends in Cognitive Sciences*, *12*(4), 163.

Marchiori, D., & Papies, E. K. (2014). A brief mindfulness intervention reduces unhealthy eating when hungry, but not the portion size effect. *Appetite, 75*, 40–45.

Moore, A., Gruber, T., Derose, J., & Malinowski, P. (2012). Regular, brief mindfulness meditation practice improves electrophysiological markers of attentional control. *Frontiers in Human Neuroscience, 6*, 18.

O'Reilly, G. A., Cook, L., Spruijt-Metz, D., & Black, D. S. (2014). Mindfulness-based interventions for obesity-related eating behaviours: A literature review. *Obesity Reviews, 15*(6), 453–461.

Ostafin, B. D., Bauer, C., & Myxter, P. (2012). Mindfulness decouples the relation between automatic alcohol motivation and heavy drinking. *Journal of Social & Clinical Psychology, 31*(7), 729–745.

Ostafin, B. D., Brooks, J. J., & Laitem, M. (2014). Affective reactivity mediates an inverse relation between mindfulness and anxiety. *Mindfulness, 5*(5), 520–528.

Papies, E. K. (2016). Health goal priming as a situated intervention tool: How to benefit from nonconscious motivational routes to health behavior. *Health Psychology Review, 10*(4), 408–424.

Papies, E. K., & Barsalou, L. W. (2015). Grounding desire and motivated behavior: A theoretical framework and review of empirical evidence. In W. Hofmann & L. F. Nordgren (Eds.), *The psychology of desire* (pp. 36–60). New York: Guilford Press.

Papies, E. K., Barsalou, L. W., & Custers, R. (2012). Mindful attention prevents mindless impulses. *Social Psychological and Personality Science, 3*(3), 291–299.

Papies, E. K., Pronk, T. M., Keesman, M., & Barsalou, L. W. (2015). The benefits of simply observing: Mindful attention modulates the link between motivation and behavior. *Journal of Personality and Social Psychology, 108*(1), 148–170.

Papies, E. K., Stroebe, W., & Aarts, H. (2008). Healthy cognition: Processes of self-regulatory success in restrained eating. *Personality and Social Psychology Bulletin, 34*(9), 1290–1300.

Papies, E. K., van Winckel, M., & Keesman, M. (2016). Food-specific decentering is associated with reduced food cravings in meditators: A preliminary investigation. *Mindfulness, 7*(5), 1123–1131.

Pidgeon, A., Lacota, K., & Champion, J. (2012). The moderating effects of mindfulness on psychological distress and emotional eating behaviour. *Australian Psychologist, 48*(4), 262–269.

Rogojanski, J., Vettese, L. C., & Antony, M. M. (2011). Coping with cigarette cravings: Comparison of suppression versus mindfulness-based strategies. *Mindfulness, 2*(1), 14–26.

Ruscio, A. C., Muench, C., Brede, E., & Waters, A. J. (2015). Effect of brief mindfulness practice on self-reported affect, craving, and smoking: A pilot randomized controlled trial using ecological momentary assessment. *Nicotine & Tobacco Research, 18*(1), 64–73.

Schoenmakers, T. M., de Bruin, M., Lux, I. F. M., Goertz, A. G., Van Kerkhof, D. H. A. T., & Wiers, R. W. (2010). Clinical effectiveness of attentional bias modification training in abstinent alcoholic patients. *Drug and Alcohol Dependence, 109*(1–3), 30–36.

Sedlmeier, P., Eberth, J., Schwarz, M., Zimmermann, D., Haarig, F., Jaeger, S., & Kunze, S. (2012). The psychological effects of meditation: A meta-analysis. *Psychological Bulletin, 138*(6), 1139–1171.

Shapiro, S. L., Carlson, L. E., Astin, J. A., & Freedman, B. (2006). Mechanisms of mindfulness. *Journal of Clinical Psychology, 62*(3), 373–386.

van der Wal, R. C., & van Dillen, L. F. (2013). Leaving a flat taste in your mouth: Task load reduces taste perception. *Psychological Science, 24*(7), 1277–1284.

Versluis, I., & Papies, E. K. (2016). Eating less from bigger packs: Preventing the pack size effect with diet primes. *Appetite, 100*, 70–79.

Wanden-Berghe, R. G., Sanz-Valero, J., & Wanden-Berghe, C. (2010). The application of mindfulness to eating disorders treatment: A systematic review. *Eating Disorders, 19*(1), 34–48.

Ward, A., & Mann, T. (2000). Don't mind if I do: Disinhibited eating under cognitive load. *Journal of Personality and Social Psychology, 78*(4), 753–763.

Webb, T. L., & Sheeran, P. (2006, March). Does changing behavioral intentions engender behavior change? A meta-analysis of the experimental evidence. *Psychological Bulletin*, *132*(2), 249–268.

Witkiewitz, K., Marlatt, G. A., & Walker, D. (2005). Mindfulness-based relapse prevention for alcohol and substance use disorders. *Journal of Cognitive Psychotherapy*, *19*(3), 211–228.

Zeidan, F., Johnson, S. K., Diamond, B. J., David, Z., & Goolkasian, P. (2010). Mindfulness meditation improves cognition: Evidence of brief mental training. *Consciousness and Cognition*, *19*(2), 597–605.

8

MINDFUL PRESENCE

Its functions and consequences in romantic relationships

Johan C. Karremans and Gesa Kappen

> When you love someone, the best thing you can offer is your presence.
> – Thich Nhat Hanh

Why are romantic partners not always able to act lovingly toward each other, even in cases of strong mutual love and commitment? Why do many relationships get challenged by regular periods of relationship distress? Why may a marriage, despite initial satisfaction, eventually end in break up, as is the case for about thirty to fifty percent of all marriages in most Western societies? Much of the history of relationship science has been concerned with these questions, trying to understand what factors contribute to romantic relationship well-being and stability, and what factors undermine it – and for good reason, as the ability to maintain a healthy functioning long-term romantic relationship can have a significant impact on an individual's psychological and physical well-being (e.g. Robles, Slatcher, Trombello, & McGinn, 2014).

While much progress has been made in understanding some of the key mechanisms that distinguish good from bad relationships (for an overview, see for example Noller & Feeney, 2013), in this chapter we suggest that research on mindfulness in relationships could provide novel insights into the reasons underlying relationship success and failure, and may extend current theoretical models of romantic relationship functioning. We define *mindfulness* here as the state of consciousness in which an individual is paying attention to current moment experiences – including feelings, thoughts, impulses, and bodily sensations – while observing these experiences with an open and accepting stance (Bishop et al., 2004). While mindfulness may affect romantic relationship functioning in several ways (e.g. Atkinson, 2013; Karremans, Schellekens, & Kappen, 2015), in this chapter we focus on one specific potential mechanism. We argue that mindful attention may promote relationship functioning by inducing awareness of relationship-threatening impulses and feelings that may otherwise escape consciousness. We will discuss the potential functions and consequences of present moment awareness, and why it may be important for relationship well-being.

Mindfulness and romantic relationships: initial evidence and prominent explanations

The scientific literature on mindfulness has left little doubt that practicing mindfulness – paying open and receptive attention to current experiences – can benefit individual well-being in various ways, ranging from less rumination and better coping with distress, and increases in subjective happiness, to better cognitive functioning (see Elkins-Brown, Teper, & Inzlicht, Chapter 5 in this volume; Leary & Diebels, Chapter 4 in this volume; Papies, Chapter 7 in this volume; Slutsky, Rahl, Lindsay, & Creswell, Chapter 6 in this volume). Indeed, a growing number of research findings suggest that mindfulness has the potential to improve the quality of people's lives on an *intra*-individual level (e.g. Brown & Ryan, 2003).

Yet, although various scholars have proposed that mindfulness can create love, compassion, and better relationships more generally, very little scientific research has examined the role of mindfulness in relationships directly, and only a handful of studies has examined its role in romantic relationships in particular. One of the first studies on this topic (Carson, Carson, Gil, & Baucom, 2004; see also Carson, Carson, Gil, & Baucom, 2007) examined the effects of a mindfulness-based relationship-enhancement intervention, which was an adapted version of the eight-week mindfulness-based stress reduction (MBSR) program, specifically adjusted to cope with distress in relationships. The studies found that couples who took part in this program, compared to a waiting list control group, reported higher levels of relationship satisfaction, closeness, and acceptance of the partner, both immediately after the intervention as well as three months later. Barnes and colleagues (Barnes, Brown, Krusemark, Campbell, & Rogge, 2007) invited romantic couples to their laboratory to discuss a recent conflict, and found that trait mindfulness was associated with lower levels of experienced negative emotions, and more positive perceptions of the partner after the conflict discussion. Also, they found that trait mindfulness was positively associated with relationship satisfaction, a correlation that has been found in several other studies (Jones, Welton, Oliver, & Thorburn, 2011; Wachs & Cordova, 2007). Although each of these studies has important limitations (e.g. reliance on self-report mindfulness; internal validity concerns inherently related to intervention studies), they have provided preliminary but consistent support in line with the notion that mindfulness may promote romantic relationship functioning.

Why may these effects occur? Before presenting our central argumentation concerning the role of present-moment awareness, we discuss two mechanisms that have been proposed most prominently. First, mindfulness promotes empathy and compassion, which in turn affects the well-being of a relationship positively (e.g. Atkinson, 2013; Kozlowski, 2013; Parker, Nelson, Epel, & Siegel, 2015). Mindful attention to current experiences is supposed to give better insight into the nature of one's own reactions and behaviour, thereby facilitating one's understanding of other people's behaviour, and increasing one's willingness to take another person's perspective (see also Condon, Chapter 9 in this volume). Moreover, it has been suggested that mindfulness practice is associated with structural changes in brain areas that facilitate empathy (e.g. Atkinson, 2013; Lucas, 2012). In line with this reasoning, various studies have found an association between trait mindfulness and empathy (e.g. Dekeyser, Raes, Leijssen, Leysen, & Dewulf, 2008), and some studies have found that mindfulness training can result in heightened levels of empathic perspective taking (Birnie, Speca, & Carlson, 2010; Shapiro, Schwartz, & Bonner, 1998; see Block-Lerner et al., 2007 for an overview). Increased empathic abilities could promote relationship well-being in several ways. For example, empathy tends to promote support-giving (Davis & Oathout, 1987), interpersonal forgiveness in the wake of conflict (McCullough, Worthington Jr., & Rachal, 1997), and the ability to accurately identify the partner's emotions and thoughts (i.e. empathic accuracy; Simpson, Ickes, & Blackstone, 1995) – all of which are factors that affect romantic relationship functioning and stability positively.

A second prominent account concerns the role of attachment in linking mindfulness to romantic relationship functioning. In fact, various scholars have argued that mindfulness and secure attachment go hand in hand (e.g. Parker, Nelson, Epel, & Siegel, 2015; Shaver, Lavy, Saron, & Mikulincer, 2007), and several studies indeed have found that trait mindfulness and attachment security are positively correlated (e.g. Pepping, Davis, & O'Donovan, 2013). Why may secure attachment and the capacity to attend mindfully to current moment experiences be associated? The lack of secure attachment representations, which is rooted in earlier relationship experiences, often is related to automatic and dysfunctional coping strategies, such as avoiding and being inattentive to stressful experiences, or becoming overwhelmed by distressing experiences (e.g. Brennan, Clark, & Shaver, 1998; Cooper, Shaver, & Collins, 1998; Shaver et al., 2007). In contrast, general feelings of safety associated with secure attachment may form a powerful resource and basis upon which to face rather than avoid or suppress difficulties and distress, and to attend to them with an open and accepting stance. Put differently, secure attachment allows an individual to respond more mindfully to current experiences, even when these experiences are threatening. Importantly, whereas secure attachment may form a basis for mindfulness, conversely, mindfulness may buffer the detrimental effects of attachment insecurity. Consistent with this reasoning, a longitudinal study by Saavedra, Chapman, and Rogge (2010) demonstrated that the negative impact of attachment anxiety on relationship satisfaction was diminished among romantic partners high in trait mindfulness. Thus, mindfulness may offer an 'alternative' strategy to cope with distressing relationship episodes, particularly among partners who are insecurely attached (cf. Cordon, Brown, & Gibson, 2009).

Surely, increased empathy and compassion, and improved coping with attachment difficulties, both may be important factors in explaining the potential role of mindfulness in romantic relationships, and examining these processes more closely provides a promising route to a better understanding of this topic. At the same time, mindfulness is not unique in promoting empathy and compassion, nor is it unique in promoting the ability to cope with attachment difficulties. To give some examples, Long and colleagues (1999; see also McCullough et al., 1997) demonstrated that empathy can be trained directly by encouraging partners to take each others' perspectives, resulting in long-term relationship benefits. Moreover, previous research has indicated that the cultivation and expression of gratitude creates interpersonal connection and empathy, and increases perceived relationship quality in both recipient and benefactor (Algoe, Gable, & Maisel, 2010; Algoe, Haidt, & Gable, 2008; McCullough, Kilpatrick, Emmons, & Larson, 2001). Likewise, several studies suggest that prayer can boost relationship satisfaction (Beach, Fincham, Hurt, McNair, & Stanley, 2008; Fincham, Lambert, & Beach, 2010), in part because it promotes empathy and attachment security (Jankowski & Sandage, 2011). Finally, some studies have shown that even repeated priming of security can bolster a sense of attachment security and promote relationship health accordingly (Mikulincer & Shaver, 2007). Thus, like mindfulness, there are various other factors that could promote compassion, empathy, and secure attachment.

The problem of *mindlessness*

Given these various possibilities to preserve and boost relationships, one may wonder why a romantic relationship would 'need' mindfulness. What is unique about mindfulness and its potential in promoting relationship functioning and stability? At its core, mindfulness is about attention, and more specifically, about directing non-judgemental attention to emotions, thoughts, bodily sensations, and impulses or action tendencies that arise in the *present* moment. We propose that many problems in romantic relationships can be traced down to the flipside of mindful presence: *mindlessness*. It is only natural and inevitable that potentially relationship-threatening situations arise: conflict occurs, external stressors are present, attractive alternative partners may show up, and so on. These situations are not problems per se, but they may evoke impulses, emotions, and thoughts that potentially threaten the relationship. We use the term *relationship threat* very broadly to refer to any experience that may undermine relationship satisfaction – either temporarily or in the longer run. Whether relationship functioning is actually threatened in these circumstances largely depends on how partners deal with these experiences, and ultimately depends on the partners' actual behavioural responses toward each other. When potentially relationship-destructive impulses or feelings escape conscious awareness, they are likely to unconsciously and automatically affect relationship-destructive responses. Indeed, the past two decades of research in psychology have demonstrated that our behaviour is often, and some would argue most of the times, guided by unconscious processes (see Wyer, 2014).

We give an example to illustrate this point, and why it can be problematic in relationships. Larry and Barbara, who have been in a romantic relationship for many years, have a dispute about their finances during dinner. They talk it over, and the argument seemingly ends there. Later that night, when Barbara sits down close to Larry on the couch, he withdraws, and Barbara feels rejected. Unbeknownst to Larry, his withdrawal behaviour is automatically guided by residual negative feelings about their dispute earlier that evening. He is, however, not consciously aware of these implicit feelings, or perhaps he has been trying to suppress them. Why is this important? When such lingering feelings are avoided or suppressed, sooner or later they are likely to leak out during an interaction, in this case resulting in withdrawal behaviour, which may induce a further sequence of negative interactions (Downey, Freitas, Michaelis, & Khouri, 1998). Potentially relationship-threatening feelings and corresponding behavioural impulses not only may be directly associated with the partner (i.e. associated with something that the partner did or said), but they may also emerge from events external to the relationship (Neff & Karney, 2004). Partners may avoid or suppress negative feelings about something that happened at their job; they may try to avoid or suppress stressful experiences related to child raising or finances; or they may avoid feelings of insecurity or ego-threat more generally. In each of these instances, when not aware of these feelings, or when trying to suppress or avoid them, they may colour responses to their partner automatically, often in an unwanted manner. Thus, in short, mind*less*ness allows potentially relationship-threatening experiences to guide responses to a partner unconsciously, resulting in relationship distress.

Mindful presence: its potential functions in romantic relationships

Now let's consider what could happen when a partner mindfully attends to feelings and impulses that potentially threaten relationship well-being. That is, what happens when a partner is *present*, paying conscious attention with an open and accepting stance to current moment experiences? A general outcome would be that mindful attention creates increased *awareness* of current-moment feelings and impulses. Thus, one may become aware of current-moment feelings, thoughts, and impulses that otherwise may have remained outside of awareness. Indeed, there is some initial evidence to suggest that mindfulness promotes awareness of otherwise unconscious feelings and responses (e.g. Brown & Ryan, 2003). We suggest that relationship success for an important part may hinge on the ability to recognize and monitor relationship-threatening impulses and feelings – noticing them *when* they arise and *while* they are present. Based on previous theorizing and some initial empirical findings (see Karremans, Schellekens, & Kappen, 2015), we propose that mindful attention and the awareness it brings to impulses and feelings may result in a number of related outcomes that could benefit romantic relationship functioning. Specifically, as we discuss in the remainder of this chapter, we propose that mindfulness may promote (1) emotional attenuation and (2) constructive communication, and may (3) facilitate the activation of motivational and regulatory resources.

Emotional attenuation

Mindfully attending to one's feelings, thoughts, or impulses, and being able to identify and recognize them, in and of itself may be a process that could regulate the intensity of distressed feelings. Research by Lieberman and colleagues (2007; Creswell, Way, Eisenberger, & Lieberman, 2007) demonstrated that attending to and labelling one's feelings in response to distressing stimuli reduces emotional reactivity (as indicated by reductions in amygdala activation). In a similar vein, Brown, Goodman, and Inzlicht (2012) found that trait mindfulness was associated with attenuated neural responses to unpleasant stimuli. These findings suggest that, in the context of a romantic relationship, mindfully observing one's inner experiences, simply identifying them, and perhaps expressing them verbally ("there is tension" or "there is anger") may take the edge off distressing feelings and desires. This may help partners to channel their anger or even aggressive impulses in the heat of an argument, and it may help them to effectively cope with other types of distress, internal or external to the relationship.

How this attenuation effect exactly may work is a topic of debate (for an extensive discussion, see Hölzel, Lazar, Gard, Schuman-Olivier, Vago, & Ott, 2011). Possibly, such attenuation effects occur in a very similar manner as exposure effects in clinical therapy. Facing rather than suppressing or avoiding the negative emotion could result in an extinction process that promotes less emotion reactivity. A related explanation is that increased frequency of giving attention in a mindful and *decentered* manner to current experiences could give an individual better insight into the transient nature of experiences (Bishop et al., 2004; Lebois et al., 2015). When one frequently gives full attention to current experiences, one may be more likely to realize that emotions and impulses arise, but also that they decline *naturally*: Feelings, thoughts, and impulses – negative or positive – come and go. Once this insight is internalized, awareness of negative experiences reduces the often natural tendency to become distressed about having negative experiences. Instead of fuelling the negative feelings or thoughts with additional reactions (e.g. negative thoughts about the negative feelings or thoughts), the negative experience naturally dissipates. This may have important implications for how partners cope with distressing experiences in their relationship. For example, awareness of negative feelings toward the partner, or about the relationship, may be more easily faced and accepted as temporary relationship distress, and less likely to be fuelled with meta-cognitive responses about these negative feelings ("Is this the partner I want to be with?"; for a discussion, see Karremans et al., 2015). Thus, giving mindful awareness to negative feelings, and being present with them without reacting to them, may attenuate negative feelings, thoughts, and impulses, or at least may prevent fuelling them.

Communication

Becoming consciously aware of otherwise implicit or unconscious feelings, and being able to identify them, is a prerequisite for verbally and explicitly communicating about them. For example, an upcoming stressful task at the workplace may be associated with implicit and perhaps suppressed feelings of insecurity, which might negatively affect behaviour toward the partner, a process often referred to as *stress spillover effects* (e.g. Neff & Karney, 2004). Outside of the individual's control, feelings of insecurity may be expressed in habitual withdrawal patterns or other negative irritable responses to the partner (Burgoon, Berger, & Waldron, 2000). However, when giving mindful attention to current moment experiences, such feelings may be more likely to enter conscious awareness. Supporting this view, findings by Brown and Ryan (2003) suggest that individuals high in trait mindfulness do have better access to implicit feelings. Only when aware of them can the individual articulate his or her feelings of insecurity, which is likely to enhance understanding in the other partner, and would promote support-giving (cf. Simpson, Rholes, & Nelligan, 1992). Similarly, negative implicit feelings toward the partner, for instance in the wake of conflict or for other reasons, are likely to be unwittingly expressed in non-verbal and destructive ways when unattended or suppressed. Again, becoming consciously aware of them seems a necessity to explicitly communicate about these feelings. Of course, whether verbal expression of these feelings will promote or undermine relationship well-being depends on the level of constructive versus destructive communication (e.g. Feeney, 1994). The point is that, if they remain unnoticed, implicit negative feelings or impulses are likely to affect responses to the partner negatively, and mindful awareness and communication may be one way in which this process may be interrupted. In support of this reasoning, Wachs and Cordova (2007) found that the association between trait mindfulness and relationship satisfaction was fully mediated by partners' ability to identify and communicate about their emotions. Similarly, Barnes and colleagues (2007) found that self-reported levels of state mindfulness were positively correlated with more constructive communication styles during a conflict discussion with the partner.

Activating motivational and regulatory resources

A common misunderstanding about mindfulness is that a mindful person may no longer experience negative (or positive) emotions. However, a mindful person obviously may experience negative emotions or thoughts about the relationship, including anger, jealousy, frustration, or distress about the relationship more generally. Also, self-interested impulses may arise that potentially threaten the relationship: Partners simply may have goals or desires that are incompatible with the well-being of the partner or relationship, they may feel an urge to retaliate when offended, or they may be tempted by attractive alternative partners. Being aware of such potentially relationship-threatening impulses and emotions does not imply that they do not occur, or that they vanish suddenly. While mindfulness can be relationship-protective because it fosters attenuation and communication, particularly intense thoughts, feelings, or impulses may require further regulation attempts.

In addition to the processes discussed earlier (i.e. attenuation and communication), we suggest that mindful awareness provides an opportunity to 'activate' motivation and regulatory resources to down-regulate relationship-threatening responses. How may this occur? The past decade has paid much theoretical and empirical attention to the question of how partners deal with and protect their relationship from relationship-threatening feelings and impulses. In general, a distinction can be made between two broad classes of factors that have been highlighted: motivational and capacity factors. First of all, a partner who is *motivated* to maintain the relationship will be more likely to engage in relationship-protective behaviour. For example, partners who report high levels of commitment to the relationship are more likely to forgive a partner (Finkel, Rusbult, Kumashiro, & Hannon, 2002). Also, they are more likely to derogate attractive alternatives, and are more likely to – quite literally – divert their attention away from alternative partners, which both can be effective strategies for resisting the temptation of attractive alternatives (Miller, 1997; Simpson, Gangestad, & Lerma, 1990). Simply put, partners who *want* to protect their relationship are more likely to do so by refraining from responses that are driven by relationship-threatening feelings or impulses.

Second, relationship protection is not just a matter of motivation, but also depends on self-regulatory *capacity* (Karremans, Pronk, & Van der Wal, 2015; Lydon & Karremans, 2015; Pronk & Righetti, 2015). Various studies have demonstrated that high self-regulation capacity helps partners to regulate and inhibit relationship-threatening impulses. For example, research findings indicate that individual differences in executive control, as well as self-reported levels of self-control, are related to successful inhibition of retaliatory feelings and impulses, and more forgiveness, in the wake of an offense (Finkel & Campbell, 2001; Pronk, Karremans, Overbeek, Vermulst, & Wigboldus, 2010). Also, when the situation constrains self-regulatory resources, or when a person is dispositionally low in self-regulation, romantically involved partners tend to display less relationship-protective responses when confronted with attractive alternative partners (Pronk, Karremans, & Wigboldus, 2011; Ritter, Karremans, & Van Schie, 2010). Together, these research findings have led researchers to conclude that both *motivation* and regulatory *capacity* are the two essential ingredients to protect an ongoing relationship: If relationship-threatening feelings, thoughts, and impulses arise, high relationship motivation and high self-regulatory capacity prevent them from actually driving behaviour (see Karremans et al., 2017).

We suggest, however, that an important aspect has been missing in this analysis: the role of awareness. As noted earlier, partners' responses may be automatically and unconsciously guided by relationship-threatening feelings, impulses and desires. Importantly, when this occurs, the route from implicit feelings and impulses to behaviour is likely to bypass any potential influence of relationship commitment or self-regulatory capacity. That is, even when the level of relationship commitment is high, and even when the level of regulatory ability is high, in a mindless state implicit feelings and impulses are behind the steering wheel of behaviour, turning relationship-threatening feelings and impulses directly into outward responses toward the partner. Yet, as noted by Hofmann and Van Dillen (2012), the role of implicit feelings and impulses in driving behaviour changes entirely as an individual becomes consciously aware of them. When impulses, desires, or implicit feelings become part of conscious experience, this "has the potential to broadcast its message to a wide range of participating systems" (Hofmann & Van Dillen, 2012; p. 319; see also Barsalou, Chapter 3 in this volume). Applying this notion to the role of mindfulness in romantic relationships, conscious awareness of relationship-threatening feelings and impulses would allow a partner to access long-term relationship motivation and goals, self-regulatory capacity, and possibly other resources (e.g. social or personal norms) that may prevent relationship-threatening feelings and impulses from directing behaviour. Again, present-moment awareness gives the partner some choice to act differently, based on broader considerations and using self-regulatory resources. Thus, we suggest that in a mind*less* state, when relationship-threatening feelings and impulses are automatically and unconsciously guiding responses toward the partner, relationship motivation and regulatory capacity may become fairly useless. Paying mindful attention to current-moment experiences should increase awareness of current impulses and feelings, thereby facilitating the detection of relationship-threat, and promoting relationship-protective behaviour. In this manner, mindfulness allows the individual to interfere in the automatic process and regulate the response.

Discussion

Back to our central questions: Why does a romantic relationship need mindfulness? Why does a relationship need present-moment awareness? As we have argued in this chapter, present-moment awareness may be a springboard to constructive and considerate responses that are likely to benefit a romantic relationship in several ways. In sum, we have suggested that mindful attention to current experiences may result in a number of potential relationship-protective outcomes: Attending to current-moment experiences may attenuate those experiences; it may promote identification of and communication about negative feelings, worries, or distress; and it could promote behaviour control because it allows the activation of motivational and self-regulatory resources. We suggest that an important topic for relationship researchers to consider is the amount of experiential awareness of relationship-threatening emotions, thoughts, and impulses, and how this may affect relationship functioning. This question has not received much theoretical attention so far, but seems a key issue in understanding why otherwise healthy relationships may fall prey to habitual dysfunctional patterns of responding.

There is some evidence that mindfulness indeed may result in relationship-protective responses in the face of relationship-threatening feelings or impulses. Several studies have demonstrated that mindfulness is associated with forgiving tendencies, suggesting that mindful awareness may help an individual to regulate negative and retaliatory responses toward an offending partner (e.g. Johns, Allen, & Gordon, 2015; Oman, Shapiro, Thoresen, Plante, & Flinders, 2008). Moreover, as noted, mindfulness has been associated with lower displays of aggression, negativity, and distress during partner conflict (Barnes et al., 2007; Hertz, Laurent, & Laurent, 2014). Papies and colleagues (2015) demonstrated that, in a sample of heterosexual participants, attending to attractive opposite-sex others with mindful attention (via a brief mindful attention induction) reduced the link between sexual motivation and perceived attractiveness. This suggests that awareness of sexual impulses toward attractive alternatives may attenuate the impulses, or that it may give a partner more opportunity to down-regulate them. Together, such findings add some credence to the claim that mindfulness may promote relationship-protective responding. However, future studies should test more directly whether present awareness of experiences results in the kind of processes we have proposed here (attenuation, identification and communication, and activating regulatory resources), and how these processes, in turn, may affect relationship protective responses in romantic couples.

It is important to note that we are not suggesting that automatic and mindless responding necessarily or always is a bad thing in a romantic relationship. In fact, as a relationship progresses over time, interaction patterns are likely to become habitualized, and it could be argued that the quality of a relationship relies, for an important part, on both partners' ability to respond to each other in a relatively effortless and automatic fashion (e.g. Kammrath et al., 2015; McNulty & Olson, 2015). Yet, in times when partners are facing distress, or when they experience negative emotions and thoughts concerning the partner or the relationship, automaticity and mindless responding may result in negative responses to each other. It is particularly in these distressing circumstances that mindful awareness of experiences may buffer the relationship against decline due to otherwise habitual and dysfunctional responding. Put differently, distressing times are likely to trigger negative cycles of relationship distress, and we suggest that mindfulness may be particularly helpful in preventing such downward cycles.

As we have noted previously (Karremans et al., 2017), mindfulness does not act as a magic wand, turning every romantic relationship into a wonderfully happy one. We propose that mindful awareness may serve a valuable function in promoting relationship functioning and satisfaction through the processes described here *if* there is a deeper basis of mutual love and commitment to the partner and the relationship. Mindful awareness allows a partner to bring his or her actions more strongly in line with his or her love and commitment to the partner. Examining such potential moderators and boundary conditions of the possible beneficial role of mindfulness in romantic relationships is a crucial area for future studies.

In addition to informing theory about romantic relationships, the potentially important role of mindful awareness in romantic relationships may be of significant practical value. As reviewed by Alberts (Chapter 2 in this volume), mindfulness can be successfully trained and cultivated, most notably by means of meditation-based intervention programs. So far, surprisingly little attention has been paid to the basic question whether the *training* of the skill to be mindful – for example, through meditation or participation in an MBSR – indeed affects romantic relationship functioning. An interesting question is whether the training of mindfulness in partner A would positively affect partner A's relationship satisfaction, and whether such effects would extend to how partner B perceives and evaluates the relationship. Also, the integration of mindfulness in existing couple therapy programs is a promising area to explore (Karremans et al., 2017). Mindfulness may be a very effective background skill from which to cultivate more specific relationship skills, such as constructive communication and conflict resolution styles.

In addition to the topics we have addressed in this chapter, many other interesting and important questions regarding the relationship between mindfulness and romantic relationship well-being remain (for a more detailed discussion of the following questions, see Karremans et al., 2017). First, our argumentation is based on the assumption that in every relationship potentially relationship-threatening feelings and impulses do arise every now and then. An additional question is whether mindfulness may be associated with lower frequency and/or intensity of threatening impulses and feelings in the first place (cf. Papies, Barsalou, & Custers, 2012). Second, does mindfulness always promote relationship well-being? For example, may mindfulness interrupt automaticity of habitual *functional* interaction patterns? Third, is mindfulness, or the lack thereof, contagious between romantic relationship partners? Fourth, and very importantly, does partner A's level of mindfulness affect outcomes for partner B? We propose that, ultimately, studying mindfulness in relationships requires researchers to take a dyadic approach. Fifth, to what extent can the positive effects of mindfulness on *individual* well-being, the focus of mindfulness research so far, be attributed to improved interpersonal functioning? Such questions have the potential to inspire many new lines of research in the forthcoming years.

Closing remarks

Research on the link between mindfulness and romantic relationships has only just begun, and scientific data should reveal whether there is an empirical basis for our theorizing. Studying this topic requires bridging two research fields, and would benefit from close collaboration between mindfulness and relationship researchers. Some scholars even have argued that examining mindfulness requires the researcher to gain first-hand experience with the concept, through meditation or for example, by participating in an MBSR program (Grossman, 2008). In any case, interdisciplinary teamwork, conceptual clarity, and also the exchange of methods between fields will be essential to study this topic systematically and thoroughly.

References

Algoe, S. B., Gable, S. L., & Maisel, N. C. (2010). It's the little things: Everyday gratitude as a booster shot for romantic relationships. *Personal Relationships, 17*(2), 217–233.

Algoe, S. B., Haidt, J., & Gable, S. L. (2008). Beyond reciprocity: Gratitude and relationships in everyday life. *Emotion, 8*(3), 425–429.

Atkinson, B. J. (2013). Mindfulness training and the cultivation of secure, satisfying couple relationships. *Couple and Family Psychology: Research and Practice, 2*(2), 73–94.

Barnes, S., Brown, K. W., Krusemark, E., Campbell, W. K., & Rogge, R. D. (2007). The role of mindfulness in romantic relationship satisfaction and responses to relationship stress. *Journal of Marital and Family Therapy, 33*(4), 482–500.

Beach, S. R., Fincham, F. D., Hurt, T. R., McNair, L. M., & Stanley, S. M. (2008). Prayer and marital intervention: A conceptual framework. *Journal of Social and Clinical Psychology, 27*(7), 641–669.

Birnie, K., Speca, M., & Carlson, L. E. (2010). Exploring self-compassion and empathy in the context of mindfulness-based stress reduction (MBSR). *Stress and Health, 26*(5), 359–371.

Bishop, S. R., Lau, M., Shapiro, S., Carlson, L., Anderson, N. D., Carmody, J., . . . Devins, G. (2004). Mindfulness: A proposed operational definition. *Clinical psychology: Science and practice, 11*(3), 230–241.

Block-Lerner, J., Adair, C., Plumb, J. C., Rhatigan, D. L., & Orsillo, S. M. (2007). The case for mindfulness-based approaches in the cultivation of empathy: Does nonjudgmental, present-moment awareness increase capacity for perspective-taking and empathic concern? *Journal of Marital and Family Therapy, 33*(4), 501–516.

Brennan, K. A., Clark, C. L., & Shaver, P. R. (1998). Self-report measurement of adult attachment: An integrative overview. In J. A. Simpson & W. S. Rholes (Eds.), *Attachment theory and close relationships* (pp. 46–76). New York: Guilford Press.

Brown, K. W., Goodman, R. J., & Inzlicht, M. (2012). Dispositional mindfulness and the attenuation of neural responses to emotional stimuli. *Social Cognitive and Affective Neuroscience, 8*, 93–99.

Brown, K. W., & Ryan, R. M. (2003). The benefits of being present: Mindfulness and its role in psychological well-being. *Journal of Personality and Social Psychology, 84*(4), 822–848.

Burgoon, J. K., Berger, C. R., & Waldron, V. R. (2000). Mindfulness and interpersonal communication. *Journal of Social Issues, 56*(1), 105–127.

Carson, J. W., Carson, K. M., Gil, K. M., & Baucom, D. H. (2004). Mindfulness-based relationship enhancement. *Behavior Therapy, 35*(3), 471–494.

Carson, J. W., Carson, K. M., Gil, K. M., & Baucom, D. H. (2007). Self-expansion as a mediator of relationship improvements in a mindfulness intervention. *Journal of Marital and Family Therapy, 33*(4), 517–528.

Cooper, M. L., Shaver, P. R., & Collins, N. L. (1998). Attachment styles, emotion regulation, and adjustment in adolescence. *Journal of personality and social psychology, 74*(5), 1380–1397.

Cordon, S. L., Brown, K. W., & Gibson, P. R. (2009). The role of mindfulness-based stress reduction on perceived stress: Preliminary evidence for the moderating role of attachment style. *Journal of Cognitive Psychotherapy, 23*(3), 258–269.

Creswell, J. D., Way, B. M., Eisenberger, N. I., & Lieberman, M. D. (2007). Neural correlates of dispositional mindfulness during affect labeling. *Psychosomatic Medicine, 69*(6), 560–565.

Davis, M. H., & Oathout, H. A. (1987). Maintenance of satisfaction in romantic relationships: Empathy and relational competence. *Journal of Personality and Social Psychology, 53*(2), 397–410.

Dekeyser, M., Raes, F., Leijssen, M., Leysen, S., & Dewulf, D. (2008). Mindfulness skills and interpersonal behaviour. *Personality and Individual Differences, 44*(5), 1235–1245.

Downey, G., Freitas, A. L., Michaelis, B., & Khouri, H. (1998). The self-fulfilling prophecy in close relationships: Rejection sensitivity and rejection by romantic partners. *Journal of Personality and Social Psychology, 75*(2), 545–560.

Feeney, J. A. (1994). Attachment style, communication patterns, and satisfaction across the life cycle of marriage. *Personal Relationships, 1*(4), 333–348.

Fincham, F. D., Lambert, N. M., & Beach, S. R. (2010). Faith and unfaithfulness: Can praying for your partner reduce infidelity? *Journal of Personality and Social Psychology, 99*(4), 649–659.

Finkel, E. J., & Campbell, W. K. (2001). Self-control and accommodation in close relationships: An interdependence analysis. *Journal of Personality and Social Psychology, 81*(2), 263–277.

Finkel, E. J., Rusbult, C. E., Kumashiro, M., & Hannon, P. A. (2002). Dealing with betrayal in close relationships: Does commitment promote forgiveness? *Journal of Personality and Social Psychology, 82*(6), 956–974.

Grossman, P. (2008). On measuring mindfulness in psychosomatic and psychological research. *Journal of Psychosomatic Research, 64*, 405–408.

Hertz, R. M., Laurent, H. K., & Laurent, S. M. (2014). Attachment mediates effects of trait mindfulness on stress responses to conflict. *Mindfulness, 6,* 483–489.

Hofmann, W., & Van Dillen, L. (2012). Desire: The new hot spot in self-control research. *Current Directions in Psychological Science, 21*(5), 317–322.

Hölzel, B. K., Lazar, S. W., Gard, T., Schuman-Olivier, Z., Vago, D. R., & Ott, U. (2011). How does mindfulness meditation work? Proposing mechanisms of action from a conceptual and neural perspective. *Perspectives on Psychological Science, 6*(6), 537–559.

Jankowski, P. J., & Sandage, S. J. (2011). Meditative prayer, hope, adult attachment, and forgiveness: A proposed model. *Psychology of Religion and Spirituality, 3*(2), 115.

Johns, K. N., Allen, E. S., & Gordon, K. C. (2015). The relationship between mindfulness and forgiveness of infidelity. *Mindfulness, 6*(6), 1462–1471.

Jones, K. C., Welton, S. R., Oliver, T. C., & Thorburn, J. W. (2011). Mindfulness, spousal attachment, and marital satisfaction: A mediated model. *The Family Journal, 19*, 357–361.

Kammrath, L. K., Peetz, J., Hara, K., Demarco, A., Wood, K., Kirkconnell, J., . . . Allen, T. (2015). It's a matter of time: The effect of depletion on communal action in romantic relationships is moderated by relationship length. *Journal of Personality and Social Psychology, 109*(2), 276–291.

Karremans, J. C., Pronk, T. M., & Van der Wal, R. C. (2015). Executive control and relationship maintenance processes: An empirical overview and theoretical integration. *Social and Personality Psychology Compass, 9*(7), 333–347.

Karremans, J. C., Schellekens, M., & Kappen, G. (2017). Bridging the sciences of mindfulness and romantic relationships a theoretical model and research agenda. *Personality and Social Psychology Review, 21*, 29–49.

Kozlowski, A. (2013). Mindful mating: Exploring the connection between mindfulness and relationship satisfaction. *Sexual and Relationship Therapy, 28*(1–2), 92–104.

Lebois, L. A., Papies, E. K., Gopinath, K., Cabanban, R., Quigley, K. S., Krishnamurthy, V., . . . & Barsalou, L. W. (2015). A shift in perspective: Decentering through mindful attention to imagined stressful events. *Neuropsychologia, 75*, 505–524.

Lieberman, M. D., Eisenberger, N. I., Crockett, M. J., Tom, S. M., Pfeifer, J. H., & Way, B. M. (2007). Putting feelings into words: Affect labeling disrupts amygdala activity in response to affective stimuli. *Psychological Science, 18*(5), 421–428.

Long, E. C., Angera, J. J., Carter, S. J., Nakamoto, M., & Kalso, M. (1999). Understanding the one you love: A longitudinal assessment of an empathy training program for couples in romantic relationships. *Family Relations, 48,* 235–242.

Lucas, M. (2012). *Rewire your brain for love: Creating vibrant relationships using the science of mindfulness.* Hay House.

Lydon, J., & Karremans, J. C. (2015). Relationship regulation in the face of eye candy: A motivated cognition framework for understanding responses to attractive alternatives. *Current Opinion in Psychology, 1,* 76–80.

McCullough, M. E., Kilpatrick, S. D., Emmons, R. A., & Larson, D. B. (2001). Is gratitude a moral affect? *Psychological Bulletin, 127*(2), 249.

McCullough, M. E., Worthington, E. L., Jr., & Rachal, K. C. (1997). Interpersonal forgiving in close relationships. *Journal of personality and social psychology, 73*(2), 321–336.

McNulty, J. K., & Olson, M. A. (2015). Integrating automatic processes into theories of relationships. *Current Opinion in Psychology, 1,* 107–112.

Mikulincer, M., & Shaver, P. R. (2007). Boosting attachment security to promote mental health, prosocial values, and inter-group tolerance. *Psychological Inquiry, 18*(3), 139–156.

Miller, R. S. (1997). Inattentive and contented: Relationship commitment and attention to alternatives. *Journal of Personality and Social Psychology, 73*(4), 758–766.

Neff, L. A., & Karney, B. R. (2004). How does context affect intimate relationships? Linking external stress and cognitive processes within marriage. *Personality and Social Psychology Bulletin, 30*(2), 134–148.

Noller, P., & Feeney, J. A. (Eds.). (2013). *Close relationships: Functions, forms and processes.* New York: Psychology Press.

Oman, D., Shapiro, S. L., Thoresen, C. E., Plante, T. G., & Flinders, T. (2008). Meditation lowers stress and supports forgiveness among college students: A randomized controlled trial. *Journal of American College Health, 56*(5), 569–578.

Papies, E. K., Barsalou, L. W., & Custers, R. (2012). Mindful attention prevents mindless impulses. *Social Psychological and Personality Science, 3*(3), 291–299.

Papies, E. K., Pronk, T. M., Keesman, M., & Barsalou, L. W. (2015). The benefits of simply observing: Mindful attention modulates the link between motivation and behavior. *Journal of Personality and Social Psychology, 108*(1), 148–170.

Parker, S. C., Nelson, B. W., Epel, E. S., & Siegel, D. J. (2015). The science of presence. In K. W. Brown, J. D. Creswell, & R. M. Ryan (Eds.), *Handbook of mindfulness: Theory, research, and practice* (pp. 225–244), New York: Guilford.

Pepping, C. A., Davis, P. J., & O'Donovan, A. (2013). Individual differences in attachment and dispositional mindfulness: The mediating role of emotion regulation. *Personality and Individual Differences, 54*(3), 453–456.

Pronk, T. M., Karremans, J. C., Overbeek, G., Vermulst, A. A., & Wigboldus, D. H. (2010). What it takes to forgive: When and why executive functioning facilitates forgiveness. *Journal of Personality and Social Psychology, 98*(1), 119.

Pronk, T. M., Karremans, J. C., & Wigboldus, D. H. (2011). How can you resist? Executive control helps romantically involved individuals to stay faithful. *Journal of Personality and Social Psychology, 100*(5), 827–837.

Pronk, T. M., & Righetti, F. (2015). How executive control promotes happy relationships and a well-balanced life. *Current Opinion in Psychology, 1,* 14–17.

Ritter, S. M., Karremans, J. C., & van Schie, H. T. (2010). The role of self-regulation in derogating attractive alternatives. *Journal of Experimental Social Psychology, 46*(4), 631–637.

Robles, T. F., Slatcher, R. B., Trombello, J. M., & McGinn, M. M. (2014). Marital quality and health: A meta-analytic review. *Psychological Bulletin, 140*(1), 140–187.

Saavedra, M. C., Chapman, K. E., & Rogge, R. D. (2010). Clarifying links between attachment and relationship quality: Hostile conflict and mindfulness as moderators. *Journal of Family Psychology, 24*(4), 380–390.

Shapiro, S. L., Schwartz, G. E., & Bonner, G. (1998). Effects of mindfulness-based stress reduction on medical and premedical students. *Journal of Behavioral Medicine*, *21*(6), 581–599.

Shaver, P. R., Lavy, S., Saron, C. D., & Mikulincer, M. (2007). Social foundations of the capacity for mindfulness: An attachment perspective. *Psychological Inquiry*, *18*(4), 264–271.

Simpson, J. A., Gangestad, S. W., & Lerma, M. (1990). Perception of physical attractiveness: Mechanisms involved in the maintenance of romantic relationships. *Journal of Personality and Social Psychology*, *59*(6), 1192–1201.

Simpson, J. A., Ickes, W., & Blackstone, T. (1995). When the head protects the heart: Empathic accuracy in dating relationships. *Journal of Personality and Social Psychology*, *69*(4), 629–641.

Simpson, J. A., Rholes, W. S., & Nelligan, J. S. (1992). Support seeking and support giving within couples in an anxiety-provoking situation: The role of attachment styles. *Journal of Personality and Social Psychology*, *62*(3), 434–446.

Wachs, K., & Cordova, J. V. (2007). Mindful relating: Exploring mindfulness and emotion repertoires in intimate relationships. *Journal of Marital and Family therapy*, *33*(4), 464–481.

Wyer, R. S. (2014). *The automaticity of everyday life: Advances in social cognition* (Vol. 10). New York: Psychology Press.

9

MINDFULNESS, COMPASSION, AND PROSOCIAL BEHAVIOUR

Paul Condon

Historically, the cultivation of mindfulness is intertwined with virtues such as compassion, love, and wisdom. Buddhist traditions evolved through philosophical argumentation that resulted in detailed understandings of the mind and contemplative practices to promote relief from suffering. The cultivation of virtuous mental states, such as compassion, was a central goal of many contemplative practices. While the scientific discourse surrounding mindfulness has acknowledged the importance of prosocial, virtuous qualities (Davidson & Harrington, 2002), early scientific work did not empirically examine such qualities, instead focusing on the cognitive benefits, neural correlates, and health outcomes associated with mindfulness (see Davidson, 2010, for a review).

The relationship between mindfulness and compassion has gained substantial interest in recent years within a growing debate about mindfulness and ethics. According to various Buddhist scholars, mindfulness originally had ethical connotations, but this has not been emphasized in modern contexts (e.g. Gethin, 2011). Modern conceptualizations of mindfulness emphasize an ethically *neutral* orientation, suggesting that the endorsement of a particular ethical framework would be inappropriate in clinical and secular contexts, instead leaving ethics as a matter of personal choice (Monteiro, Musten, & Compson, 2015). Yet an ethically neutral approach could lead to problematic applications of mindfulness-based training. Mindfulness practice motivated by personal gain or self-improvement, for example, could fertilize the self-centred processes that are thought to contribute to one's own chronic dissatisfaction (i.e. greed, hatred, and delusion; Gethin, 1998). The question of ethics has thus raised concerns about the fidelity of modern applications of mindfulness in secular settings.

Contemporary psychological literature characterizes mindfulness as present-cantered and non-judgemental (e.g. Kabat-Zinn, 2011) whereas certain Buddhist styles of mindfulness involve the discrimination of virtuous and non-virtuous mental states, suggesting a possible divergence between contemporary and traditional perspectives. In the traditional view, the ability to observe and define mental content allows the practitioner to relate experience to a system of mental states distinguished as virtuous and non-virtuous (i.e. the Abhidharma; Bodhi, 2011). In this sense, "right mindfulness" includes discrimination about mental qualities, intentions, and the conviction to engage in purposeful action. This approach is contrasted with the contemporary notion of mindfulness as *non-judgemental* awareness (Kabat-Zinn, 2011). Scholars have thus questioned whether modern mindfulness-based interventions that lack an ethical framework merely provide symptomatic relief rather than insight into the roots of suffering (Monteiro, Musten, & Compson, 2015).

In light of the debate about ethics in mindfulness, some Buddhist scholars have traced the origins of non-judgemental awareness to Buddhist sources. In particular, the concept of non-judgemental awareness appears to stem from a category of *non-dual* meditation practices that view mental states as absent of subject-object duality (Dunne, 2015). From this *non-dual* perspective, all mental states are constructions or representations, independent of the desirability of the content of a mental state (i.e. virtuous vs. non-virtuous). The non-dual style of mindfulness merely witnesses the arising and falling of mental states, leading to the insight that all states are mental representations, rather than reflections of an objective reality. This approach appears to have had direct influence on the style of practice found in contemporary mindfulness programs (Dunne, 2015; Kabat-Zinn, 2011). Nevertheless, non-dual traditions assume that the success of these practices is dependent on the allegiance to an ethical code in one's lifestyle (Dunne, 2015). As such, ethics could play a key role in promoting benefits associated with mindfulness. The empirical study of mindfulness and virtuous outcomes remains of great interest.

Social psychology is uniquely positioned to evaluate the role of mindfulness and meditation in promoting virtuous outcomes. Social psychology is known for its theoretical and methodological innovations for measuring social processes and behaviour in settings that reflect the world in which people live. Moreover, virtuous states and behaviours most often occur in social and relational contexts (see also Karremans & Kappen, Chapter 8 in this volume). Hence, social psychological methods offer an ideal approach to test the causal influence of mindfulness on compassion and prosocial behaviour. This chapter will review the current scientific research investigating the impact of mindfulness and related meditation techniques on compassion and prosocial behaviour, and identify open questions for future research.

Defining mindfulness

A thorough exploration of mindfulness constructs is beyond the scope of this chapter (for review, see Karremans & Papies, Chapter 1 in this volume); however, one definitional issue is germane to the present chapter. The Buddhist traditions that inspired contemporary mindfulness interventions do not offer a unified or authoritative account of mindfulness, leading to confusion in the psychological literature about what exactly mindfulness is (Dunne, 2011, 2015; Gethin, 2011; Lutz, Jha, Dunne, & Saron, 2015;). Instead, Buddhist scholars have suggested that "mindfulness" represents a family of related but divergent practices and skills (Dunne, 2015; Gethin, 2011; Lutz et al., 2015). One perspective, for example, differentiates mindfulness practices that aim to calm and focus the mind (e.g. focused attention, Lutz, Slagter, Dunne, & Davidson, 2008) and enhance the ability to monitor activity of the mind (e.g. open monitoring, Lutz et al., 2008). These skills are trained in programs such as mindfulness-based stress reduction (MBSR; Kabat-Zinn, 2011), but they are also featured in programs related to compassion- and loving-kindness meditation (LKM).

A variety of meditation programs draw from distinct but related mindfulness- and compassion-based contemplative models (Lavelle Heineberg, 2016). In the history of the modern mindfulness movement, dating to Jon Kabat-Zinn's introduction of the MBSR program, the emphasis on compassion was often implicit, through language encouraging a "non-judgemental" and "accepting" approach to one's own negative emotional states, which is thought to create a compassionate context or frame (Dunne, 2015). More recently, however, compassion has become explicitly thematized in secular mindfulness programs, such as the mindful self-compassion program (MSC; Neff & Germer, 2013). In addition, mindfulness skills are often the initial elements of programs that explicitly state compassion as a primary goal (e.g. cognitive-based compassion training [CBCT]; sustainable compassion training [SCT], Heineberg, 2016). Mindfulness is not an isolated skill, but is often developed in the context of additional contemplative techniques that directly emphasize compassion.

Defining compassion

Historically, the term *compassion* has been used interchangeably with terms such as *empathy*, *empathic concern*, and *sympathy* (e.g. Wispé, 1986). Yet many authors now differentiate *compassion* from *empathy*. Empathy typically refers to processes that allow an individual to understand another person's mental state, either through perspective-taking (also called "cognitive empathy", "theory of mind", "mental state attribution", or "mentalizing") or through emotional contagion (also called "affective empathy", or "experience sharing") (Zaki & Ochsner, 2012). Compassion can be differentiated from empathy based on the motivations that underlie one's resonance with another's mental state. Here, compassion is defined as an other-oriented emotional state that arises in response to another's suffering and motivates one to alleviate another's suffering (Goetz, Keltner, & Simon-Thomas, 2010). A large body of research suggests that other-oriented states of compassion increase the likelihood of prosocial behaviour (e.g. Batson, 2011). In the following section, I review empirical evidence that links mindfulness, compassion, and prosocial action.

Empirical investigations of mindfulness, compassion, and prosocial action

Researchers in social psychology and related disciplines have demonstrated that a variety of mindfulness and related meditation interventions increase compassionate states and prosocial behaviours. Many of these studies examined the impact of meditation curricula that included explicit aspirations related to love and compassion (e.g. LKM, compassion meditation). In the following section, I review the impact of various meditation-based programs to provide a sense of the literature as a whole.

Self-reported effects of meditation

Many studies have examined the impact of mindfulness, loving-kindness, or compassion training on self-reported compassion and social connection. Experimental studies have demonstrated that mindfulness training resulted in increased self-reports in empathy and compassion, for example, among medical students completing the MBSR curriculum (Shapiro, Schwartz, & Bonner, 1998) and middle-aged adults completing the Mindful Self-Compassion curriculum (Neff & Germer, 2013). Elsewhere, MBSR resulted in increased self-reported self-compassion, but not other-oriented compassion following training (Birnie, Speca, & Carlson, 2010). Some studies have also reported strong correlations between self-reported dispositional mindfulness and empathy and compassion (Cameron & Fredrickson, 2015; Dekeyser, Raes, Leijssen, Leysen, & Dewulf, 2008). Compassion and loving-kindness training also produced increases in self-reported compassion (Jazaieri et al., 2013, 2015; Sahdra et al., 2011; Wallmark, Safarzadeh, Daukantaite, & Maddux, 2013).

In a notable series of studies, Fredrickson and colleagues (Fredrickson, Cohn, Coffey, Pek, & Finkel, 2008; Kok et al., 2013) demonstrated that 6 weeks of LKM, compared with a wait-list control, increased daily self-reported positive emotions throughout training (Fredrickson et al., 2008; Kok et al., 2013). Furthermore, these increases in positive emotion accounted for increases in a variety of personal resources, including self-reported positive relations with others and perceived social connection (Fredrickson et al., 2008; Kok et al., 2013). These studies provided initial evidence that meditation might increase qualities related to compassion and prosocial action. Nevertheless, scientists are well-aware of the need to move beyond measures that rely on self-report, especially in the domain of mindfulness, where self-report measures are likely to conflate achievement with aspiration (Grossman & Van Dam, 2011; see also Alberts, Chapter 2 in this volume). Thus, despite the encouraging results described earlier, it remained an open question as to whether mindfulness and meditation-related practices produce changes in social behaviour. To move beyond self-report, a number of researchers have investigated the neural underpinnings of meditation.

Neural effects of meditation

A number of neuroimaging studies have examined the neural effects of long-term and short-term meditation training. One notable study compared the effects of 8 weeks of training in mindfulness, compassion, or an active control group on participants' reactivity during non-meditative states after the course (Desbordes et al., 2012). Among participants with no prior meditation experience, those completing mindfulness training exhibited decreased amygdala response to people in negative settings whereas those completing compassion meditation exhibited increased right-amygdala responses to negative images. This work provides strong evidence that mindfulness and compassion meditation alters neural responses to others, even in a non-meditative ordinary state independent of experimenter instructions. These findings are also consistent with a growing number of studies showing the effects of compassion meditation on empathic reactivity to others' suffering (Klimecki, Leiberg, Lamm, & Singer, 2013; Klimecki, Leiberg, Ricard, & Singer, 2014; Lutz, Brefczynski-Lewis, Johnstone, & Davidson, 2008; Mascaro, Rilling, Tenzin Negi, & Raison, 2013; Weng et al., 2013). Collectively, these studies provide compelling evidence that relatively brief training in mindfulness and other forms of meditation increase one's ability to identify another's suffering, but here again, it remained unclear whether neural effects would translate to actual social behaviour. Methods from social psychology and behavioural economics have helped move this line of investigation forward.

Behavioural effects of meditation

A number of studies have employed behavioural measures to indirectly assess compassion and prosocial action resulting from mindfulness training. Indirect measures used to assess prosocial tendencies in the meditation literature have included non-verbal behaviours indicating affiliation, interest, or a lack of hostility toward one's spouse (Kemeny et al., 2012), and expressions of sadness in reaction to others' suffering (Rosenberg et al., 2015). These studies demonstrated that short-term training in mindfulness enhanced outcomes that could be indicative of prosocial motivation (i.e. non-verbal behaviours).

To move beyond indirect measures of compassion and prosocial action, researchers have employed tasks from behavioural economics to examine the effects of meditation training on generosity in monetary transactions. Various studies across laboratories have demonstrated that LKM enhances prosocial behaviour in computer-based video games (Leiberg, Klimecki, & Singer, 2011) and online economic transactions (Weng, Fox, Hessenthaler, Stodola, & Davidson, 2015; Weng et al., 2013). A mindfulness-based kindness curriculum resulted in more donation of stickers among preschool-age children to peers (Flook, Goldberg, Pinger, & Davidson, 2015). Of greatest interest, the neural effects of compassion training predicted increased altruistic behaviour in an economic transaction (Weng et al., 2013). Though it remained unclear as to what extent economic generosity would extend to real-world situations involving the suffering of another individual, these findings are encouraging of the role of meditation in promoting prosocial behaviour.

Social psychological methods that model real-world scenarios offer the ability to overcome the limitations of self-report and demand characteristics. Through such an approach, researchers can employ measures of prosocial action when participants themselves are not aware that they are being observed. In an effort to link mindfulness and compassion training to prosocial action, my team constructed a paradigm designed to reduce demand by measuring behaviours outside of the laboratory context. Specifically, we examined whether participants helped a stranger in pain following training in a meditation curriculum compared with those in a control group (Condon, Desbordes, Miller, & DeSteno, 2013).

To construct a real-world measure of prosocial behaviour in response to another's pain, we utilized confederates (i.e. actors and actresses ostensibly participating in research studies) to expose participants to the suffering of another individual outside the laboratory. Prior to the participant's arrival, two female confederates sat in a designated waiting area possessing three chairs. Upon arriving at the waiting area, the participant sat in the last remaining chair. A third female confederate then appeared with crutches and a large walking boot. She visibly winced while walking, stopped just as she arrived at the chairs, then audibly sighed in discomfort, and leaned back against a wall. The sitting confederates remained seated and did not acknowledge the presence of the crutch confederate or the participant. To assess prosocial action, we measured whether the true participant offered his or her seat to the suffering confederate, despite the inaction of the sitting confederates. This scenario constitutes a classic "bystander" situation, in which the presence of non-responsive others typically leads to a reduction in helping behaviour (Darley & Latané, 1968). In these situations, bystanders often look to each other for information about the appropriate course of action and thereby misinterpret each other's apparent lack of concern and fail to intervene (Latané & Rodin, 1969).

After 8 weeks of training in either compassion- or mindfulness-based meditation, participants offered their seat to relieve the pain of the suffering confederate at a much higher rate (50%), compared with those in a wait-list control (15%) (Condon et al., 2013). Moreover, those completing compassion and mindfulness training were equally likely to provide help, suggesting that discussions of compassion that occurred within the compassion course were not entirely responsible for producing enhanced compassionate action. As is the case with many meditation studies (see also Alberts, Chapter 2 in this volume), the nature of this design required that one group (i.e. meditators) came together for repeated classes, thereby creating a context that afforded interaction with other individuals participating in the study, which may have produced social consequences that could account for increased levels of helping behaviour relative to a wait-list control that had no possibility of such social interaction. To rule out this possibility, we measured the number of people that participants interacted with on a regular basis before and after training, using the Social Network Index (Cohen, Doyle, Skoner, Rabin, & Gwaltney, 1997). Participants in the meditation group did not experience a growth in their social network as a function of participating in an organized class. Thus, the experience of participating in a group activity was unlikely to account for our central finding.

In a second study, we replicated these findings using mindfulness trainings delivered via mobile devices through a commercially available platform ("Headspace") (Lim, Condon, & DeSteno, 2015). Following just 2 weeks of training, those completing mindfulness training via the mobile app demonstrated an increased rate of prosocial responding to the confederate in need (37%) compared with those in the active control group (14%). Importantly, the relative level of prosocial action in the active control group matched that of the wait-list control group (16%) from the first study (Condon et al., 2013), suggesting that the 23% increase in helping among meditating participants represents an increase from baseline.

Taken together, these results provided evidence that compassion and mindfulness meditation can enhance prosocial responding in real-world settings, even in a situation that is known to reduce prosocial action. In both studies, meditation training removed the impact of non-responsive bystanders, yielding helping rates that approximate those found in conditions with no bystanders present (Latané & Nida, 1981). Moreover, participation in a meditation class in a gathering of peers did not appear to account for the effect. Those who trained in mindfulness via a smartphone application did not practice with peers or a caring teacher in a social setting, yet still exhibited an increased rate of prosocial responding compared with an active control group.

In summary, this body of research demonstrates that mindfulness and related practices can increase compassion and prosocial action. However, this literature spans different types of meditation and mindfulness curricula. In turn, we do not know whether – or to what extent – various elements of mindfulness account for increases in compassion and prosocial action. Going forward, a major challenge for the field will involve isolating the active ingredients that account for these effects. In the following section, I speculate on mechanisms that might explain the relationship between mindfulness, compassion, and prosocial action.

Mechanisms of mindfulness

A number of factors have been conceptualized as mechanisms that explain how mindfulness produces various cognitive and emotional benefits (e.g. Hölzel et al., 2011; Lutz et al., 2015), many of which may be relevant to interpersonal behaviours and one's readiness to help others in need. Three mechanisms appear particularly relevant. One of the most common elements of mindfulness includes the capacity to regulate and sustain attention on a given object for a sustained period of time, often called *focused attention* meditation or *śamatha* (Lutz et al., 2008). As part of training in focused attention, the practitioner is encouraged to calmly notice when the mind wanders and simply return attention to the selected object. A number of studies have empirically demonstrated that mindfulness-based meditation does increase attention capacities (e.g. Slagter et al., 2007; Tang et al., 2007). In social contexts, enhanced attention capacities may increase the ability to attend to the needs of others, thereby increasing the likelihood that one would recognize an opportunity or need to engage in action to help others.

A second crucial mindfulness-induced mechanism is heightened body awareness, which includes the ability to notice subtle fluctuations in bodily sensations (Hölzel et al., 2011; see also Elkins-Brown, Teper, & Inzlicht, Chapter 5 in this volume). Awareness of the body is a central target of many Buddhist traditions, perhaps because the ability to ground subjective experience in the activity of the body may represent one avenue to insight into the transient nature of phenomena (Farb et al., 2015;

Hölzel et al., 2011; Lutz et al., 2015). In the psychological and neuroscience literature, awareness of bodily sensations, also referred to as *interoceptive awareness,* may play a key role in awareness of emotional experience (e.g. Craig, 2003), thereby guiding decision-making and self-regulation. Although behavioural data suggest that meditation may not increase awareness of bodily sensations, neuroscience evidence is suggestive that meditation training does increase activity in the insula (Farb et al., 2007), a brain region involved in interoceptive awareness (Craig, 2003). Moreover, the insula is also involved in processing others' emotional experiences and information related to risk and uncertainty (see Singer, Critchley, & Preuschoff, 2009 for a review). In social scenarios, heightened awareness of one's own bodily processes may also increase empathic processing, increasing the likelihood that one may act to help others.

A third mechanism that appears promising to explain the link between mindfulness, compassion, and prosocial action is that of dereification, a capacity that all styles of mindfulness meditation train (Lutz et al., 2015; see also Papies, Chapter 7 in this volume). Lutz and colleagues defined *dereification* as "the degree to which thoughts, feelings, and perceptions are phenomenally interpreted as mental processes rather than as accurate depictions of reality" (Lutz et al., 2015, p. 639).[1] As Lutz and colleagues describe, high reification occurs when thoughts are taken to be real, as if the object or situation described by the thought is occurring in the present moment. For example, reification occurs in a state of rumination when the thought "I am a failure" appears to represent an accurate description of the self, and as a consequence, depressed mood and negative affect is enhanced (Lutz et al., 2015). However, with dereification, thoughts are experienced simply as mental events in a field of sensory, affective, and somatic feeling tones. Through dereification, one can engage flexibly with thoughts without reifying any of them as the only perspective on a situation. One potential result is higher cognitive flexibility, including outcomes such as creative problem solving and perspective-taking (Colzato, Ozturk, & Hommel, 2012).

A subtype of dereification includes what some have referred to as changes in perspectives on the self (Hölzel et al., 2011; Lutz et al., 2015). In Buddhist traditions, fixation on a particular identity or narrative about an autonomous, enduring self is a key contributor to afflictive motivations and desires, such as greed and aversion. As such, many contemplative practices are designed to deconstruct the self (Dahl, Lutz, & Davidson, 2015; Hölzel et al., 2011). From a contemplative perspective, deconstructing the self appears to be one important avenue that allows for opening up to the experiences of others, engaging in perspective-taking, and experiencing compassion (see also Leary & Diebels, Chapter 4 in this volume). Dereification may also explain the prosocial effects of mindfulness by promoting emotion-regulation capacities. By experiencing emotions as representations, dereification engendered by mindfulness may reduce negative affect (Krishnakumar & Robinson, 2015) and automatic, reactive responses (see also Barsalou, Chapter 3 in this volume). Consistent with this view, mindfulness may increase compassion by reducing automatic aversion to others' suffering. A recent experimental study examined participants' facial expressions in reaction to others' suffering and found that meditators did not exhibit aversive facial expressions to others' suffering, compared with those in a wait-list control (Rosenberg et al., 2015).

Mechanisms of mindfulness in bystander contexts

The review of mindfulness mechanisms raises questions about how they could help overcome social pressures that typically reduce helping in bystander contexts. We can develop a number of hypotheses regarding how mindfulness-based mediators might reduce the bystander effect and enhance prosocial actions despite the inaction of others. Classic social psychological theory and research postulated a number of processes that interfere with helping in bystander contexts (Latané & Darley, 1970), which could be modulated by mindfulness-based mechanisms. Three processes in particular interfere with helping behaviour when other bystanders are present. First, *social influence* refers to the process by which people look to others as sources of information when faced with an ambiguous situation. In bystander scenarios, it may be unclear whether another individual is in need. Thus, people look to others to determine the appropriate course of action, notice that no one is moving to help the person in need, and thereby decide not to help. The collective outcome of non-intervention has also been called "pluralistic ignorance" (Latané & Darley, 1970). As reviewed earlier, mindfulness may increase the relevance of another's suffering through attention regulation and body awareness. Through enhanced attentional capacities, mindfulness may simply make people more aware of another's suffering, thereby reducing the ambiguity of the situation. In our hallway scenario, for example, it may be that mindfulness increases the capacity to notice the individual in need, notice subtle expressions of suffering, and engage in action to help. Enhanced body awareness may also increase prosocial action by increasing empathic awareness of another's suffering, thereby reducing the ambiguity of the situation, leading to reduced reliance on the social environment to determine the correct course of action.

The second process that reduces helping in bystander contexts is *audience inhibition* or *evaluation apprehension* (Latané & Darley, 1970). Bystander situations incur a high risk of embarrassment because the potential helper's actions could be viewed and evaluated in a negative manner by the bystanders or the victim. People not only look to others for the appropriate course of action, but also fear embarrassment of acting in such a way that may violate social norms or annoy the target in need of help. In fact, negative social evaluation is a robust cause of subjective and physical stress (Dickerson, Mycek, & Zaldivar, 2008). In the hallway scenario reported earlier, participants might believe it would be impolite to offer the seat to the confederate on crutches. Mindfulness may reduce evaluation apprehension through dereification and its impact on the self-concept. As such, participants may be less likely to reify narratives about the self that would be targeted in social evaluations. In line with this perspective, prosocial action and cooperation appears to be an intuitive action (Rand et al., 2014). Dereification of the self may yield more confidence to act in a decisive manner despite inaction of others. In fact, in our paradigm, most participants who offer their seat to the suffering confederate do so within 15 seconds.

Finally, the third process that interferes with helping is *diffusion of responsibility* (Latané & Darley, 1970). When others are present in a helping scenario, the potential costs to the self of not acting, such as threats to one's reputation, are reduced. Any given individual will bear less responsibility for not acting because there were also other individuals in the context who did not help. The costs for not acting are therefore spread out among a number of individuals, reducing the likelihood that any given individual will come to aid. To the extent that mindfulness meditation promotes a deconstruction of the self, via dereification, it may also promote greater willingness and readiness to take on the responsibility to help others. Enhanced empathic processing via body awareness may also increase the likelihood of experiencing compassion and thereby taking personal responsibility for action.

In addition to bystander situations, mindfulness might increase compassion and prosocial responses to others across various contexts. Through enhanced cognitive flexibility generated by dereification, for example, one may be able to entertain social targets as more than one's current representation. For example, while simulating the memory of a difficult co-worker, the thought "He's a jerk" might occur. In a moment of high reification, the thought of the other person as a jerk is taken to represent an accurate depiction of the other, as if that is the other's true nature or identity. However, through dereification, one can come to entertain alternative conceptualizations of the co-worker, including the possibility of the deeper humanity of the other, who has similar desires to experience happiness and reduce suffering. This process is one of the crucial capacities trained in explicit compassion-based training protocols such as CBCT and SCT (Heineberg, 2016). In this way, dereification may explain recent findings that meditation training reduces implicit bias toward out-group members (Kang, Gray, & Dovidio, 2014; Lueke & Gibson, 2015; see also Berry & Brown, Chapter 11 in this volume). The process of dereification applied to one's own self-concept may also explain findings that individual differences in self-reported non-attachment predict prosocial behaviour as rated by peers (Sahdra, Ciarrochi, Parker, Marshall, & Heaven, 2015).

Laboratory studies that use simple manipulations may be particularly effective in isolating active ingredients and mechanisms responsible for psychological change and positive social outcomes (see also Alberts, Chapter 2 in this volume). Recent work, for example, used laboratory-based instructions to investigate the process of dereification on responses to images of desirable food. Results indicated that simple instruction resulted in the ability to overcome impulsive reactions to desirable food (Papies, Barsalou, & Custers, 2012; see also Papies, Chapter 7 in this volume). A similar laboratory-based approach could lead to insight about the elements of mindfulness that produce prosocial outcomes.

In this vein, a recent study employed a brief laboratory-based mindfulness induction and examined its effects on empathic accuracy and prosocial action (Tan, Lo, & Macrae, 2014). Participants listened to a 5-minute mindfulness manipulation, with instructions to facilitate focused attention on the breath and awareness of mind-wandering (such instructions could promote attention regulation, body awareness, and dereification to some degree). Participants then completed tasks that measured empathic accuracy and compassion. Those participants who listened to the mindfulness recording, compared with those who were simply instructed to immerse in their own thoughts and emotions, performed better on the test of empathic accuracy and demonstrated higher levels of compassion in handwritten notes to a confederate. Although the use of a short-term, low-dose mindfulness induction may never approximate the training that constitutes extended meditation practice, experimental studies such as these might prove helpful in isolating active ingredients involved in sustained contemplative training. Although this study did not isolate the exact mechanisms at play, a similar approach could be used in conjunction with measures of the relevant mechanisms.

Conclusion

In summary, meditation training in a variety of forms increases prosocial mental states and behaviour. Secularized mindfulness and compassion-based training protocols thus offer an exciting avenue to increase compassion among people interested and willing to engage in meditation practice. As the empirical investigation of meditation grows, it will be important to note similarities and differences across studies based on divergent mindfulness- and compassion-based training protocols (e.g. MBSR, MSC, CBCT, SCT). It may also be the case that personality traits or other demographic characteristics impact the manner in which a person responds to such practices. Identifying the particular challenges and benefits that different individuals experience with different practices may provide important insights on the application of these practices in clinical or educational settings.

The research reviewed in this chapter falls within an ongoing dialogue concerning the growing popularity of mindfulness and the application of meditation in various secular settings. In its original Buddhist context, meditation is accompanied by ethical intentions and spiritual goals that are considered crucial for the efficacy of meditation practice. The translation of meditation to secular contexts presents a challenge that is unlikely to always produce the outcomes that meditation practitioners hope for (e.g. compassion, happiness). Indeed, mindfulness-based mechanisms of attention regulation, body awareness, and dereification are not inherently motivational phenomena. Compassion involves the motivation to care for others and the desire to alleviate suffering. The adoption of a particular mental framework (e.g. ethical intentions) in which contemplative practice is embedded may interact with mindfulness-based mechanisms to promote compassion and prosocial action. Yet the endorsement of a Buddhist ethical context would be inappropriate in secular settings. One viable alternative could centre on the integration of mindfulness practices with discussions and activities based on the growing literature in psychology on social relations and well-being to create a prosocial, relational framework (Baer, 2015). In the end, our field awaits empirical investigations of the impact of intention and context on the downstream effects of meditation practice.

Note

1 Dereification is similar to "defusion" and "decentering" in the psychological literature. Lutz et al. (2015) noted that these terms conflate dereification and meta-awareness, which involves monitoring experience. Dereification is distinguished from meta-awareness, which can occur even in states of high reification (such as anxiety).

References

Baer, R. (2015). Ethics, values, virtues, and character strengths in mindfulness-based interventions: A psychological science perspective. *Mindfulness, 6,* 956–969.

Batson, C. D. (2011). *Altruism in humans.* New York: Oxford University Press.

Birnie, K., Speca, M., & Carlson, L. E. (2010). Exploring self-compassion and empathy in the context of Mindfulness-Based Stress Reduction (MBSR). *Stress and Health, 26,* 359–371.

Bodhi, B. (2011). What does mindfulness really mean? A canonical perspective. *Contemporary Buddhism, 12,* 19–39.

Cameron, C. D., & Fredrickson, B. L. (2015). Mindfulness facets predict helping behavior and distinct helping-related emotions. *Mindfulness, 6,* 1211–1218.

Cohen, S., Doyle, W. J., Skoner, D. P., Rabin, B. S., & Gwaltney, J. M. (1997). Social ties and susceptibility to the common cold. *Journal of the American Medical Association, 277,* 1940–1944.

Colzato, L. S., Ozturk, A., & Hommel, B. (2012). Meditate to create: The impact of focused-attention and open-monitoring training on convergent and divergent thinking. *Frontiers in Psychology, 3,* 1–5.

Condon, P., Desbordes, G., Miller, W. B., & DeSteno, D. (2013). Meditation increases compassionate responses to suffering. *Psychological Science, 24,* 2125–2127.

Craig, A. D. (2003). Interoception: the sense of the physiological condition of the body. *Current Opinion in Neurobiology, 13*(4), 500–505.

Dahl, C. J., Lutz, A., & Davidson, R. J. (2015). Reconstructing and deconstructing the self: Cognitive mechanisms in meditation practice. *Trends in Cognitive Sciences, 19,* 515–523.

Darley, J., & Latané, B. (1968). Bystander intervention in emergencies: Diffusion of responsibility. *Journal of Personality and Social Psychology, 8,* 377–383.

Davidson, R. J. (2010). Empirical explorations of mindfulness: Conceptual and methodological conundrums. *Emotion, 10,* 8–11.

Davidson, R. J. & Harrington, A. (2002). *Visions of compassion.* New York: Oxford Univeristy Press.

Dekeyser, M., Raes, F., Leijssen, M., Leysen, S., & Dewulf, D. (2008). Mindfulness skills and interpersonal behaviour. *Personality and Individual Differences, 44,* 1235–1245.

Desbordes, G., Negi, L. T., Pace, T. W. W., Wallace, B. A., Raison, C. L., & Schwartz, E. L. (2012). Effects of mindful-attention and compassion meditation training on amygdala response to emotional stimuli in an ordinary, non-meditative state. *Frontiers in Human Neuroscience, 6,* 1–15.

Dickerson, S. S., Mycek, P. J., & Zaldivar, F. (2008). Negative social evaluation, but not mere social presence, elicits cortisol responses to a laboratory stressor task. *Health Psychology: Official Journal of the Division of Health Psychology, American Psychological Association, 27,* 116–121.

Dunne, J. D. (2011). Toward an understanding of non-dual mindfulness. *Contemporary Buddhism, 12,* 71–88.

Dunne, J. D. (2015). Buddhist styles of mindfulenss: A heuristic approach. In M. D. Robinson, B. P. Meier, & B. D. Ostafin (Eds.), *Hanbook of mindfulness and self-regulation* (pp. 251–270). New York: Springer.

Farb, N., Daubenmier, J., Price, C. J., Gard, T., Kerr, C., Dunn, B. D., . . . & Mehling, W. E. (2015). Interoception, contemplative practice, and health. *Frontiers in Psychology, 6,* 763.

Farb, N. A., Segal, Z. V., Mayberg, H., Bean, J., McKeon, D., Fatima, Z., & Anderson, A. K. (2007). Attending to the present: Mindfulness meditation reveals distinct neural modes of self-reference. *Social Cognitive and Affective Neuroscience, 2*(4), 313–322.

Flook, L., Goldberg, S. B., Pinger, L., & Davidson, R. J. (2015). Promoting prosocial behavior and self-regulatory skills in preschool children through a mindfulness-based kindness curriculum. *Developmental Psychology, 51,* 44–51.

Fredrickson, B. L., Cohn, M. A., Coffey, K. A., Pek, J., & Finkel, S. M. (2008). Open hearts build lives: Positive emotions, induced through loving-kindness meditation, build consequential personal resources. *Journal of Personality and Social Psychology, 95,* 1045–1062.

Gethin, R. (1998). *The foundations of Buddhism.* New York: Oxford University Press.

Gethin, R. (2011). On some definitions of mindfulness. *Contemporary Buddhism, 12,* 263–279.

Goetz, J. L., Keltner, D., & Simon-Thomas, E. (2010). Compassion: An evolutionary analysis and empirical review. *Psychological Bulletin, 136,* 351–374.

Grossman, P., & Van Dam, N. T. (2011). Mindfulness, by any other name . . .: Trials and tribulations of sati in Western psychology and science. *Contemporary Buddhism, 12,* 219–239.

Hölzel, B. K., Lazar, S. W., Gard, T., Schuman-Olivier, Z., Vago, D. R., & Ott, U. (2011). How does mindfulness meditation work? Proposing mechanisms of action from a conceptual and neural perspective. *Perspectives on Psychological Science, 6,* 537–559.

Jazaieri, H., Jinpa, G. T., McGonigal, K., Rosenberg, E. L., Finkelstein, J., Simon-Thomas, E., . . . Goldin, P. R. (2013). Enhancing compassion: A randomized controlled trial of a compassion cultivation training program. *Journal of Happiness Studies, 14,* 1113–1126.

Jazaieri, H., Lee, I. A., McGonigal, K., Jinpa, T., Doty, J. R., Gross, J. J., & Goldin, P. R. (2015). A wandering mind is a less caring mind: Daily experience sampling during compassion meditation training. *The Journal of Positive Psychology, 9760,* 1–14.

Kabat-Zinn, J. (2011). Some reflections on the origins of MBSR, skillful means, and the trouble with maps. *Contemporary Buddhism, 12,* 281–306.

Kang, Y., Gray, J. R., & Dovidio, J. F. (2014). The nondiscriminating heart: Lovingkindness meditation training decreases implicit intergroup bias. *Journal of Experimental Psychology. General, 143,* 1306–1313.

Kemeny, M. E., Foltz, C., Cavanagh, J. F., Cullen, M., Giese-Davis, J., Jennings, P., . . . Ekman, P. (2012). Contemplative/emotion training reduces negative emotional behavior and promotes prosocial responses. *Emotion, 12,* 338–350.

Klimecki, O. M., Leiberg, S., Lamm, C., & Singer, T. (2013). Functional neural plasticity and associated changes in positive affect after compassion training. *Cerebral Cortex, 23,* 1552–1561.

Klimecki, O. M., Leiberg, S., Ricard, M., & Singer, T. (2014). Differential pattern of functional brain plasticity after compassion and empathy training. *Social Cognitive and Affective Neuroscience, 9,* 873–879.

Kok, B. E., Coffey, K. A., Cohn, M. A., Catalino, L. I., Vacharkulksemsuk, T., Algoe, S. B., . . . Fredrickson, B. L. (2013). How positive emotions build physical health: Perceived positive social connections account for the upward spiral between positive emotions and vagal tone. *Psychological Science, 24,* 1123–1132.

Krishnakumar, S., & Robinson, M. D. (2015). Maintaining an even keel: An affect-mediated model of mindfulness and hostile work behavior. *Emotion, 15*(5), 579–589.

Latané, B. & Darley, J. M. (1970). *The unresponsive bystander: Why doesn't he help?* New York: Appleton-Century-Crofts.

Latané, B., & Nida, S. (1981). Ten years of research on group size and helping. *Psychological Bulletin, 89,* 308–324.

Latané, B., & Rodin, J. (1969). A lady in distress: Inhibiting effects of friends and strangers on bystander intervention. *Journal of Experimental Social Psychology, 5,* 189–202.

Lavelle Heineberg, B. D. (2016). Promoting caring: Mindfulness-and compassion-based contemplative training for educators and students. In K. A. Schonert-Reichl & R. W. Roeser (Eds.), *Handbook of eindfulness in Education: Integrating theory and research into practice* (pp. 285–294). New York: Springer.

Leiberg, S., Klimecki, O., & Singer, T. (2011). Short-term compassion training increases prosocial behavior in a newly developed prosocial game. *PloS ONE, 6,* e17798.

Lim, D., Condon, P., & DeSteno, D. (2015). Mindfulness and compassion: An examination of mechanism and scalability. *PLoS ONE, 10,* e0118221.

Lueke, A., & Gibson, B. (2015). Mindfulness meditation reduces implicit age and race bias: The role of reduced automaticity of responding. *Social Psychological and Personality Science, 6,* 284–291.

Lutz, A., Brefczynski-Lewis, J., Johnstone, T., & Davidson, R. J. (2008). Regulation of the neural circuitry of emotion by compassion meditation: Effects of meditative expertise. *PloS ONE, 3,* e1897.

Lutz, A., Jha, A., Dunne, J. D., & Saron, C. D. (2015). Investigating the phenomenological matrix of mindfulness-related practices from a neurocognitive perspective. *American Psychologist, 70,* 632–658.

Lutz, A., Slagter, H. A., Dunne, J. D., & Davidson, R. J. (2008). Attention regulation and monitoring in meditation. *Trends in Cognitive Sciences, 12,* 163–169.

Mascaro, J. S., Rilling, J. K., Tenzin Negi, L., & Raison, C. L. (2013). Compassion meditation enhances empathic accuracy and related neural activity. *Social Cognitive and Affective Neuroscience, 8,* 48–55.

Monteiro, L. M., Musten, R. F., & Compson, J. (2015). Traditional and contemporary mindfulness: Finding the middle path in the tangle of concerns. *Mindfulness, 6,* 1–13.

Neff, K. D., & Germer, C. K. (2013). A pilot study and randomized controlled trial of the mindful self-compassion program. *Journal of Clinical Psychology, 69,* 28–44.

Papies, E., Barsalou, L., & Custers, R. (2012). Mindful attention prevents mindless impulses. *Social Psychological and Personality Science, 3,* 291–299.

Rand, D. G., Peysakhovich, A., Kraft-Todd, G. T., Newman, G. E., Wurzbacher, O., Nowak, M. A., & Greene, J. D. (2014). Social heuristics shape intuitive cooperation. *Nature Communications, 5,* 3677.

Rosenberg, E. L., Zanesco, A. P., King, B. G., Aichele, S. R., Jacobs, T. L., Bridwell, D. A., . . . Saron, C. D. (2015). Intensive meditation training influences emotional responses to suffering. *Emotion, 15,* 775–790.

Sahdra, B. K., Ciarrochi, J., Parker, P. D., Marshall, S., & Heaven, P. (2015). Empathy and non-attachment independently predict peer nominations of prosocial behavior of adolescents. *Frontiers in Psychology, 6,* 263.

Sahdra, B. K., MacLean, K. A., Ferrer, E., Shaver, P. R., Rosenberg, E. L., Jacobs, T. L., . . . Saron, C. D. (2011). Enhanced response inhibition during intensive meditation training predicts improvements in self-reported adaptive socioemotional functioning. *Emotion, 11,* 299–312.

Shapiro, S. L., Schwartz, G. E., & Bonner, G. (1998). Effects of mindfulness-based stress reduction on medical and premedical students. *Journal of Behavioral Medicine, 21,* 581–599.

Singer, T., Critchley, H. D., & Preuschoff, K. (2009). A common role of insula in feelings, empathy and uncertainty. *Trends in Cognitive Sciences, 13*(8), 334–340.

Slagter, H. A., Lutz, A., Greischar, L. L., Francis, A. D., Nieuwenhuis, S., Davis, J. M., & Davidson, R. J. (2007). Mental training affects distribution of limited brain resources. *Public Library of Science Biology, 5*(6), 138.

Tan, L. B. G., Lo, B. C. Y., & Macrae, C. N. (2014). Brief mindfulness meditation improves mental state attribution and empathizing. *PLoS ONE, 9*, e110510.

Tang, Y. Y., Ma, Y., Wang, J., Fan, Y., Feng, S., Lu, Q., . . . & Posner, M. I. (2007). Short-term meditation training improves attention and self-regulation. *Proceedings of the National Academy of Sciences, 104*(43), 17152–17156.

Wallmark, E., Safarzadeh, K., Daukantaite, D., & Maddux, R. E. (2013). Promoting altruism through meditation: An 8-week randomized controlled pilot study. *Mindfulness, 4*, 223–234.

Weng, H. Y., Fox, A. S., Hessenthaler, H. C., Stodola, D. E., & Davidson, R. J. (2015). The role of compassion in altruistic helping and punishment behavior. *PLoS ONE, 10*, e0143794.

Weng, H. Y., Fox, A. S., Shackman, A. J., Stodola, D. E., Caldwell, J. Z. K., Olson, M. C., . . . Davidson, R. J. (2013). Compassion training alters altruism and neural responses to suffering. *Psychological Science, 24*, 1171–1180.

Wispé, L. (1986). The distinction between sympathy and empathy: To call forth a concept, a word is needed. *Journal of Personality and Social Psychology, 50*, 314–321.

Zaki, J., & Ochsner, K. (2012). The neuroscience of empathy: Progress, pitfalls and promise. *Nature Neuroscience, 15*, 675–680.

10

MINDFULNESS IN EDUCATION

Enhancing academic achievement and student well-being by reducing mind-wandering

Michael D. Mrazek, Claire M. Zedelius, Madeleine E. Gross, Alissa J. Mrazek, Dawa T. Phillips, and Jonathan W. Schooler

Over the last decade, the field of social psychology has become increasingly interested in investigating the effects of mindfulness. Dozens of laboratory studies have rigorously examined the short-term outcomes of mindfulness in controlled settings, yet the lack of ecological validity in these studies means that the claims of applied value and generalizability are limited. Meanwhile, mindfulness training has been introduced into classrooms worldwide in hopes of improving academic achievement and student well-being. While evidence of the efficacy of mindfulness-based intervention programs in schools is promising, their evaluation often still lacks the methodological rigor and strong theoretical foundation of most laboratory studies on mindfulness (Weare, 2013). That is a gap that we are hoping to help close. Here, we aim to integrate the extant literature on mindfulness and educational outcomes from both controlled experiments as well as research in more naturalistic settings. By synthesizing this diverse work and reconciling strengths and weaknesses from the various approaches, we present a theoretical model of the benefits of mindfulness-based interventions in primary and secondary education for student well-being and academic achievement.

Student attentiveness is an essential basis of learning, yet high levels of distraction are widely prevalent in schools (Lindquist & McLean, 2011; Rosengrant, 2011). A primary source of distraction is mind-wandering, which is commonly defined as engaging in spontaneous task-unrelated thought (Smallwood & Schooler, 2006). Mind-wandering is rampant during lectures, class activities, and even exams, and this frequency of mind-wandering has a myriad of destructive outcomes. For example, mind-wandering during (live or recorded) lectures has been shown to be detrimental to the retention of newly learned information as well as performance on exams (Risko, Anderson, Sarwal, Engelhardt, & Kingstone, 2012; Schacter & Szpunar, 2015; Wammes, Seli, Allan, Boucher, & Smilek, 2016). Additionally, across middle and high school populations, mind-wandering while taking a reading test predicts worse reading comprehension (Mrazek, Phillips, Franklin, Broadway, & Schooler, 2013). In addition to the consequences on academic achievement and learning, students also mind-wander during class and daily life in ways that are associated with greater stress and worse mood (Mrazek, Phillips et al., 2013).

The problem of mind-wandering in the classroom is unmistakable, but solutions are less clear. Students are often asked to pay attention, but are rarely taught or trained in how to do so. As described in this chapter, our research suggests that a compounding source of frustration for students is that many of them also believe that their tendency for mind-wandering and their capacity to focus attention are immutable. To offset this, teachers attempt to retain their students' attention by strategically altering educational tools and the learning environment (Jensen, 1998; Sammons, 1995). For instance, teachers often provide activities that are sensitive to limited attention spans in order to stimulate student interest (Sylwester & Cho, 1993). Although altering educational tools and the learning environment is helpful, careful observation of almost any school classroom reveals the ongoing challenge of gaining and sustaining students' undivided attention.

As a result, mindfulness training programs have been introduced into schools, often with the hope and intention of helping students to better focus their attention over extended durations. Although promising, these training programs lack sufficient evaluation (Weare, 2013). Indeed, almost none of these programs have been specifically assessed with respect to their impact on reducing student mind-wandering, which may be one of the core mechanisms through which these interventions enhance learning (Cheyne, Solman, Carriere, & Smilek, 2009; Risko et al., 2012; Schacter & Szpunar, 2015; Schooler, Reichle, & Halpern, 2004; Wammes et al., 2016). Here we review the relevant literature and present a theoretical model that could be used to assess extant training programs as well as guide the design of potentially even more effective mindfulness curricula. In the present model, mindfulness training is proposed to reduce student mind-wandering – in part by reducing negative affect and changing students' mindsets about their mental capacities – which in turn may improve academic achievement.

Mindfulness training for wandering minds

Despite considerable disagreement regarding what the word *mindfulness* should convey, there is near consensus that sustained attentiveness, or the capacity to avoid distraction, represents an essential and valuable element. Thus, we suggest that augmenting mindfulness is a strategic route to decreasing mind-wandering. Strategies for reducing mind-wandering have immense practical significance given the robust relationship between mind-wandering and impaired task performance. Mind-wandering is a ubiquitous phenomenon that occupies approximately 30–50% of waking life (Kane et al., 2007; Killingsworth & Gilbert, 2010). This frequency is alarming, since mind-wandering is associated with impaired task vigilance (Cheyne et al., 2009), reading comprehension, and information retention

(Cheyne et al., 2009; Risko et al., 2012; Schacter & Szpunar, 2015; Schooler, Reichle, & Halpern, 2004; Smallwood, McSpadden, & Schooler, 2008; Wammes et al., 2016).

Although most of this research has been conducted with young adult samples, mind-wandering among students in grades 6–12 is also associated with impaired reading comprehension (Mrazek, Phillips et al., 2013). Mind-wandering additionally impairs performance on measures of mental aptitude – such as working memory capacity and fluid intelligence – that are predictive of academic achievement, job performance, and other practical indicators (Conway et al., 2005). In fact, nearly 50% of the shared variance among working memory capacity, fluid intelligence, and performance on the SAT is explained by the mind-wandering that occurs during these assessments (Mrazek, Smallwood, Franklin et al., 2012). The capacity to avoid mind-wandering during demanding tasks is clearly an important ability with implications for learning and academic achievement.

Mind-wandering and its disruptive effects on task performance could be reduced by interventions that increase mindfulness. After all, individuals with high trait-levels of mindfulness mind-wander less in daily life and during laboratory tasks requiring focused attention (Mrazek, Smallwood, & Schooler, 2012). Furthermore, mindfulness training improves aspects of attention closely linked to mind-wandering, including executive attention, perceptual sensitivity, and task vigilance (MacLean et al., 2010; Tang et al., 2007).

Several converging studies with adult samples suggest that mindfulness training can directly influence rates of mind-wandering. In one study, the brief practice of mindful breathing in the laboratory resulted in reduced mind-wandering during an immediately subsequent task (Mrazek, Smallwood, & Schooler, 2012). In another investigation, 2 weeks of mindfulness training decreased mind-wandering and improved working memory capacity and reading comprehension among undergraduates (Mrazek, Franklin, Phillips, Baird, & Schooler, 2013). This same pattern of reduced mind-wandering and improved performance was also found using a 6-week mindfulness-based lifestyle change program (Mrazek, Mooneyham, Mrazek, & Schooler, 2016). Similarly, 4 weeks of breath counting training has also been shown to decrease mind-wandering relative to working memory training and no training controls (Levinson, Stoll, Kindy, Merry, & Davidson, 2014). Furthermore, the impact of meditation training is not limited to self-reported mind-wandering. Zanesco et al. examined the effect of meditation training on people's capacity to notice when text intermittently became meaningless (Zanesco et al., 2016) (a measure found to closely index mind-wandering during reading [Zedelius, Protzko, & Schooler, 2016]). In two separate studies, they found that meditation training not only reduced self-reported mind-wandering but enhanced performance on this objective "gibberish detection" index of mind-wandering.

Several lines of research also suggest that mindfulness training can directly affect attention and mind-wandering among youth. Students with Attentional Deficit Hyperactivity Disorder showed reduced symptomatology after receiving mindfulness training (van de Weijer-Bergsma et al., 2011). Among incarcerated youth, a mindfulness training program buffered these adolescents from the attentional deterioration that often accompanies the high-stress interval of incarceration (Leonard et al., 2013). Ongoing research in our lab – described in greater detail later – also indicates that mindfulness training can be effective for high school students. In a recent pilot study, high school freshmen demonstrated reduced levels of mind-wandering during both a reading test as well as during daily life after receiving 4 weeks of mindfulness training and practicing on a daily basis with their teacher in the classroom (Mrazek, Phillips, & Schooler, 2015).

These results cumulatively suggest that mindfulness training holds substantial promise for alleviating the disruptive impact of mind-wandering in learning environments. The practice of mindfulness often promotes a persistent effort to regain and maintain focus on a single aspect of experience despite frequent interruptions of unrelated thoughts, perceptions, or personal concerns (Bishop et al., 2004). When this ability to concentrate is redirected to a challenging task, it can prevent the displacement of crucial task-relevant information by distractions. At least some of the performance enhancements derived from mindfulness training therefore appear to result from directly training the capacity for focused attention. However, mindfulness training may also influence mind-wandering and academic achievement indirectly by reducing levels of negative affect or by changing students' mindsets about their ability to control their attention.

Mindfulness, negative affect, and mind-wandering

Considerable research indicates that attention is influenced by negative affect. Self-reported measures of negative affect reliably predict both increased mind-wandering and reduced performance during laboratory tasks of vigilance and learning (Mrazek, Smallwood, & Schooler, 2012; Smallwood, Fishman, & Schooler, 2007). Similarly, naturally occurring episodes of mind-wandering during daily life tend to be associated with lower mood (Killingsworth & Gilbert, 2010). Furthermore, experimentally inducing negative affect increases mind-wandering, suggesting negative affect plays a causal role in the emergence of mind-wandering (Smallwood, Fitzgerald, Miles, & Phillips, 2009). This relationship between negative affect and mind-wandering extends to youth as well. Levels of negative affect as measured by the Positive and Negative Affect Schedule are associated with students' trait-levels of mind-wandering during daily life as well as their rates of mind-wandering during reading (Mrazek, Phillips et al., 2013). Specifically, adolescents who experience less positive and more negative affect on a regular basis tend to mind-wander more.

Meanwhile, one of the most reliable effects of mindfulness training for youth is reduced negative affect. Multiple studies using different samples of middle and high school students have found that mindfulness reduces negative affect, stress, and anxiety (Broderick & Metz, 2009; Elder et al., 2011; Kuyken et al., 2013). These results reinforce the numerous studies with adult samples indicating that mindfulness practice can improve mood (Hofmann, Sawyer, Witt, & Oh, 2010). In fact, studies with adult samples suggest that mindfulness training may reduce negative affect in a manner that enhances attention and working memory. Military personnel receiving mindfulness training during a highly stressful pre-deployment interval experienced less negative affect and less deterioration of working memory capacity (Jha, Stanley, Kiyonaga, Wong, & Gelfand, 2010). Similarly, teachers who received mindfulness training showed reduced depression and anxiety, as well as enhanced attention and working memory capacity (Roeser et al., 2013). This research suggests that reducing negative affect may be a key mechanism through which mindfulness affects mind-wandering and academic achievement.

Growth mindsets, mind-wandering, and academic achievement

Considerable research has demonstrated that factors relevant to academic achievement are influenced not only by a person's cognitive capacities, but also by their personal *beliefs* about their own capacities, often referred to as implicit theories, lay theories, or mindsets (e.g. Chiu, Hong, & Dweck, 1997; Dweck, Chiu, & Hong, 1995). Mindsets function as a "lens" through which people interpret information about themselves and the world around them. Even though mindsets are often implicit – that is, they are rarely explicitly articulated (Ross, 1989) – they can have powerful effects on learning and behaviour. Mindsets can influence whether people seek out or eschew challenges, what kinds of goals they set, and how they respond to setbacks or feedback (Burnette, O'Boyle, VanEpps, Pollack, & Finkel, 2013; Molden & Dweck, 2006; Robins & Pals, 2002).

A mindset that has been shown to be particularly beneficial in academic contexts is the belief that one's intelligence is malleable and can be improved with practice, rather than being genetically or otherwise determined, a system of beliefs that has been termed a *growth mindset* (Aronson, Fried, & Good, 2002; Dweck, 2006; Dweck et al., 1995). Numerous studies have shown that students with a growth mindset, compared to those who view their abilities as fixed, reach higher academic achievements (Dweck, 2006). Moreover, interventions that encouraged students to view intelligence as a skill that can be developed rather than a fixed ability led to marked improvements in students' grades and state-wide test scores (Aronson et al., 2002; Blackwell, Trzesniewski, & Dweck, 2007; Good, Aronson, & Inzlicht, 2003; Yaeger & Dweck, 2012; Yaeger & Walton, 2011).

Recent research from our laboratory has extended this research by investigating whether students hold different beliefs related to attentional control and mind-wandering, and whether these beliefs influence their ability to focus during various tasks. When noticing their mind-wandering, some people may view this as an uncontrollable event – a spontaneous attentional fluctuation inherent in the functioning of their brain. Others may view it as a failure on their part to regulate their attention. These different beliefs seem to be reflected in the way people talk about mind-wandering. A person may choose to say, "I wasn't paying attention," implying a certain level of personal control and responsibility, or phrase it more passively: "My mind was wandering."

To assess such differences in people's mindsets and examine their relation to actual mind-wandering, we developed a novel scale (building on the existing *theories of intelligence* scale by Hong, Chiu, & Dweck, 1995) that assesses the extent to which individuals believe that they have control over their tendency to mind-wander (Zedelius et al., 2016). In several studies, we found that scores on the scale varied among individuals, and predicted their self-reported ability to focus in everyday life as well as their mind-wandering frequencies during reading tasks in the laboratory. We also found that undergraduate students who tended to believe more strongly that mind-wandering is controllable showed greater reading comprehension performance, providing further evidence that mindsets related to attentional control can have important implications for academic success. Moreover, in a pilot study with 58 high school freshmen, we found that mindsets related to attentional control significantly predicted not only rates of mind-wandering during testing and levels of reading comprehension, but also trait-levels of mindfulness.

Having established the importance of theories of mind-wandering in correlational studies, we next conducted two experimental studies indicating that these mindsets can be influenced by providing explicit information suggesting that people have (or lack) reasonable control over their tendency to mind-wander (Zedelius et al., 2016). However, challenging people's mindsets about attentional control through explicit information alone may not necessarily elicit long-lasting changes. After all, the belief that one has control over one's wandering mind is easily challenged by frequent and sometimes frustrating experiences of mind-wandering in everyday life. Achieving stable improvements in mind-wandering may therefore require both an adaptive mindset as well as practices that enhance attentional control.

Many published mindfulness interventions do already include extensive didactic instruction of various mindsets related to mindfulness. An important distinction regarding control over mind-wandering that is often made in mindfulness training programs is attempting to suppress thoughts versus allowing thoughts to pass away without elaborating, judging, or analyzing them. Many mindfulness programs emphasize the importance of recognizing that thoughts arise spontaneously, and that the control one has is in choosing not to elaborate these thoughts. This suggests that mindfulness training may have nuanced effects on participants' theories of mind-wandering, though this remains a largely unexplored research question. Future work could track changes in mindsets about various dimensions of attentional control and observe how these changes relate to objective outcomes of mindfulness training. For instance, many people report being surprised at the sheer number of thoughts that rush through their mind when they first practice mindfulness, and without effective guidance this experience could lead to disempowering theory of mind-wandering as completely uncontrollable. However, with instruction and practice people may find that they can control such mental turbulence by deliberately adopting an attitude towards spontaneous thoughts that dampens their capacity to draw the mind away from the present.

A mechanistic theory of change

Although teachers and policymakers work hard to maximize student learning, students' ability to pay attention and integrate information is compromised by the pervasive tendency to mind-wander. The reviewed research suggests a theory of change regarding how mindfulness interventions – ideally complemented by additional mindset instructions – could lead to improved academic achievement. The theory begins with the premise, strongly supported by various lines of research, that mind-wandering is a crucial constraint to effective learning. When students' minds are not present in the learning environment, students are unable to extract the relevant material and learning is compromised. This initial detriment in information extraction and integration leads to a cascading process of learning difficulties, where it becomes increasingly challenging to understand and relate to new material (Smallwood et al., 2007). Students can find themselves falling further and further behind. We propose that mindfulness interventions can target the compounding disruptive effects of mind-wandering on learning in at least three ways. First, mindfulness directly strengthens the capacity to remain focused. Second, mindfulness reduces negative emotional states. Since negative affect is itself a major source of distraction, the attenuation of this aversive state enhances mental focus and helps to further minimize mind-wandering. Third, we think that mindfulness training may enhance people's general dispositions towards both a general growth mindset regarding their overall intelligence and a specific growth mindset regarding their capacity to control their wandering minds. Such changes may be the result of personal observation stemming from mindfulness practice and may be further enhanced by the supplementation of mindfulness training with additional instruction that particularly targets those mindsets. Given that our research has found that students who believe their attention is not under their control tend to mind-wander more frequently, helping students gain new perspectives on their ability to control their attention may provide an important route for minimizing mind-wandering and enhancing learning. In short, this mechanistic theory of change (see Figure 10.1) posits that mindfulness instruction increases attentional focus, reduces negative affect, and encourages adaptive mindsets, which in turn lead to reduced mind-wandering, and thereby enhance students' ability to attend to the material that they encounter in the classroom and in other learning contexts.

Although we have chosen to focus on a small set of key mechanisms that may enhance academic achievement by reducing mind-wandering, it is important to recognize that there are a number of additional ways that mindfulness training may support academic success. For instance, socially prescribed perfectionism within schools may increase distress and anxiety, which can in turn lead to burnout and lower student success (Short and Mazmanian, 2013; Walburg, 2014). Mindfulness training may protect against these negative outcomes by decreasing the ruminative thought that leads to worry, depression, and perfectionism (Burns, Lee, and Brown, 2011; Short and Mazmanian, 2013). Furthermore, emotional regulation engendered by mindfulness training not only reduces negative affect but also positively impacts

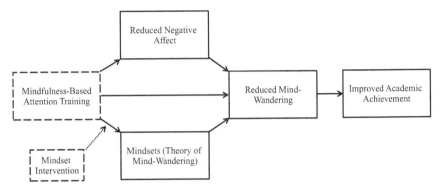

FIGURE 10.1   Theory of change

student-teacher interactions and student motivation (Graziano et al., 2007). A complete understanding of the ways that mindfulness enhances academic achievement will ultimately require a more complex model that incorporates dispositional and behavioural skills conducive to effective learning environments.

A review of the sparse literature on the benefits of mindfulness for academic achievement

Given the existing evidence that mindfulness training can improve mood, reduce mind-wandering, and change beliefs about one's control over attention, our theory of change would suggest that there should also be strong evidence that mindfulness training can enhance academic achievement. Perhaps surprisingly, relatively little research is available to speak to this question. However, the few studies that have sought such assessment have generally observed a positive impact on learning outcomes.

For instance, using standardized measures of academic performance, some research teams have observed improvements after a brief mindfulness intervention. Nidich and colleagues examined the effect of a mindfulness-based transcendental meditation (TM) program on subsequent performance on the California Standards Tests (CST), a state-wide standardized test administered to measure student progress (Nidich et al., 2011). In this study, the at-risk group of urban middle school students who completed the TM program showed a boost of at least one performance level on both math and English categories. The TM intervention has also been shown to improve graduation rates and decrease dropout rates among high school students (Colbert, 2013). Similarly, in a different mindfulness-based program, reading and science grades have likewise been found to significantly improve after participation (Bakosh, Snow, Tobias, Houlihan, & Barbosa-Leiker, 2015). Finally, after completing the mindfulness-based stress reduction (MBSR; Kabat-Zinn, 1990) program, a group of students age 16–18 performed significantly better on the General Certificate of Education (GCE), another standardized test for grade-schoolers (Bennett & Dorjee, 2015). These researchers observed a medium-sized effect in test scores differences between those who completed MBSR compared to control students. In sum, although few studies have rigorously assessed the utility of mindfulness training programs for academic achievement, the few that have point towards promising results.

Providing mindfulness training for students with learning disabilities appears to further highlight the potential this type of practice may have on learning outcomes. In addition to the benefits on academic performance, mindfulness-based programs have provided some success in improving social skills and behavioural conduct, while also reducing emotional disturbances and social difficulties (Beauchemin, Hutchins, & Patterson, 2008; Haydicky, Wiener, Badali, Milligan, & Ducharme, 2012). For instance, Beauchemin and colleagues (2008) investigated the efficacy of a mindfulness meditation intervention on adolescents with mild to severe learning disabilities. After a 5-week interval, results revealed significant improvements in social anxiety as well as academic and social skills, as measured by a subscale in the Social Skills Rating System (SSRS).

Reducing social anxiety and improving attention in the classroom are goals of researchers and educators alike, partially due to the strong role they play in predicting academic success (Boyer & Sedlacek, 1988). Specifically, a longitudinal analysis demonstrated that attention was one of the top factors affecting learning outcomes (Duncan & Magnuson, 2011). Fortunately, mindfulness training programs seem to be useful from this perspective as well. A well-established intervention, mindfulness-based cognitive therapy, recently adapted for use with children, revealed improvements in attention, managing anxiety, and curbing behavioural problems (Semple, Lee, Rosa, & Miller, 2010). Emphasizing the interplay between mental health and learning capabilities, additional research has shown the detrimental effect that anxiety can have on attention, which may be especially relevant in test anxiety situations (Bellinger, DeCaro, & Ralston, 2015; Wine, 1971). Correspondingly, a randomized controlled trial, which applied a mindfulness-based program to primary school students, found significant improvements in social skills, selective attention, and managing test anxiety (Burke, 2010).

Despite the promise of these preliminary findings, more methodologically robust research is needed to substantiate the connection between academic achievement and mindfulness training. Many of the studies reviewed here lack a large and diverse sample, which limits both the statistical power and generalizability of these results (Bennett & Dorjee, 2015; Shapiro, Brown, Thoresen, & Plante, 2011). In addition, lack of randomization and the use of teacher-based measures may introduce causal ambiguity and reporting bias, respectively (Flook, Goldberg, Pinger, & Davidson, 2015; Maynard, Solis, & Miller, 2015). The methodological weaknesses of existing investigations may be due to the nascent nature of research in this area, where feasibility has been prioritized over stringent experimental designs (Burke, 2010). For example, the paucity of rigorous research may result in part from the practical challenges of implementing large-scale randomized control trials that include waitlist or active-treatment controls in schools. Many constraints make this task difficult, including ensuring consistent delivery of the mindfulness program by teachers, gaining informed consent from guardians, and merging the programs seamlessly into the existing school curricula. Nevertheless, rigorously controlled studies are ultimately necessary for the causal inference that mindfulness training can improve academic achievement (see Alberts, Chapter 2 in this volume). Given the encouraging preliminary results and the accelerating societal interest in mindfulness, methodologically sound, large-scale investigations are a worthwhile and important future direction for the field.

Conclusion

Worldwide interest in mindfulness is growing rapidly. Mindfulness is being introduced into most every major sector of society, including education, medicine, business, government, and the military. This rapid expansion has been fuelled by the encouraging results of rigorous scientific investigation, and research into the many benefits of mindfulness continues to progress. Yet despite these encouraging trends, the role that mindfulness will play in our society's learning institutions over the long-term is at a pivotal crossroads. Despite mounting documentation of the *benefits* of mindfulness, relatively little is known about the mechanisms through which these benefits are achieved and the strategies through which mindfulness can be taught most effectively. Much more research is needed to examine the mediating (a) cognitive processes such as mind-wandering, (b) affective processes such as mood, and (c) implicit beliefs or mindsets about attentional control. To ensure that the growing demand for mindfulness can be met with high-quality evidence-based instruction, a new science of the *instruction* of mindfulness is essential. Our hope is that the theory of change presented here can provide some direction in thinking about how to optimize mindfulness training programs for youth as well as how to assess the mechanisms that might underlie potential improvements in academic achievement.

Author note

The writing of this manuscript was supported by the Institute of Education Sciences grant R305A110277, the John Templeton Foundation grant 52071, and the Shao Family Charitable Trust. The content does not necessarily reflect the position or policies of the U.S. government.

References

Aronson, J., Fried, C. B., & Good, C. (2002). Reducing the effects of stereotype threat on African American college students by shaping theories of intelligence. *Journal of Experimental Social Psychology, 38*(2), 113–125.

Bakosh, L. S., Snow, R. M., Tobias, J. M., Houlihan, J. L., & Barbosa-Leiker, C. (2015). Maximizing mindful learning: Mindful awareness intervention improves elementary school students' quarterly grades. *Mindfulness, 7,* 59–67.

Beauchemin, J., Hutchins, T. L., & Patterson, F. (2008). Mindfulness meditation may lessen anxiety, promote social skills, and improve academic performance among adolescents with learning disabilities. *Complementary Health Practice Review*, *13*(1), 34–45.

Bellinger, D. B., DeCaro, M. S., & Ralston, P. A. (2015). Mindfulness, anxiety, and high-stakes mathematics performance in the laboratory and classroom. *Consciousness and Cognition*, *37*, 123–132.

Bennett, K., & Dorjee, D. (2015). The impact of a Mindfulness-Based Stress Reduction course (MBSR) on well-being and academic attainment of sixth-form students. *Mindfulness, 7,* 105–114.

Bishop, S. R., Lau, M., Shapiro, S., Carlson, L., Anderson, N. D., Carmody, J., . . . Devins, G. (2004). Mindfulness: A proposed operational definition. *Clinical Psychology: Science and Practice*, *11*(3), 230–241. http://doi.org/10.1093/clipsy.bph077

Blackwell, L. S., Trzesniewski, K. H., & Dweck, C. S. (2007). Implicit theories of intelligence predict achievement across an adolescent transition: A longitudinal study and an intervention. *Child Development*, *78*(1), 246–263.

Boyer, S. P., & Sedlacek, W. E. (1988). Noncognitive predictors of academic success for international students: A longitudinal study. *Journal of College Student Development*, *29*(3), 218–223.

Broderick, P. C., & Metz, S. (2009). Learning to breathe: A pilot trial of a mindfulness curriculum for adolescents. *Advances in School Mental Health Promotion*, *2*(1), 35–46.

Burke, C. A. (2010). Mindfulness-based approaches with children and adolescents: A preliminary review of current research in an emergent field. *Journal of Child and Family Studies*, *19*(2), 133–144.

Burnette, J. L., O'Boyle, E. H., VanEpps, E. M., Pollack, J. M., & Finkel, E. J. (2013). Mindsets matter: A meta-analytic review of implicit theories and self-regulation. *Psychological Bulletin*, *139*(3), 655.

Burns, J. L., Lee, R. M., & Brown, L. J. (2011). The effect of meditation on self-reported measures of stress, anxiety, depression, and perfectionism in a college population. *Journal of College Student Psychotherapy*, *25*(2), 132–144.

Cheyne, A. J., Solman, G. J., Carriere, J. S., & Smilek, D. (2009). Anatomy of an error: A bidirectional state model of task engagement/disengagement and attention-related errors. *Cognition*, *111*(1), 98–113.

Chiu, C., Hong, Y., & Dweck, C. S. (1997). Lay dispositionism and implicit theories of personality. *Journal of Personality and Social Psychology*, *73*(1), 19–30.

Colbert, R. (2013). Effect of the transcendental meditation program on graduation, college acceptance and dropout rates for students attending an urban public high school. *Education*, *133*(4), 495–501.

Conway, A. R. A., Kane, M. J., Bunting, M. F., Hambrick, D. Z., Wilhelm, O., & Engle, R. W. (2005). Working memory span tasks: A methodological review and user's guide. *Psychonomic Bulletin & Review. Special Issue: Memory Strength and Recency Judgements*, *12*(5), 769–786.

Duncan, G. J., & Magnuson, K. (2011). The nature and impact of early achievement skills, attention skills, and behavior problems. In G. J. Duncan & R. J. Murnane (Eds.), *Whither Opportunity* (pp. 47–69). New York: Russell Sage.

Dweck, C. S. (2006). *Mindset: The new psychology of success*. New York. Random House Publishing Group.

Dweck, C. S., Chiu, C., & Hong, Y. (1995). Implicit theories and their role in judgments and reactions: A word from two perspectives. *Psychological Inquiry*, *6*(4), 267–285.

Elder, C., Nidich, S. Colbert, R., Hagelin, J., Grayshield, L., Oviedo-Lim, D., . . . Gerace, D. (2011). Reduced psychological distress in racial and ethnic minority students practicing the transcendental meditation program. *Journal of Instructional Psychology*, *38*(2), 109.

Flook, L., Goldberg, S. B., Pinger, L., & Davidson, R. J. (2015). Promoting prosocial behavior and self-regulatory skills in preschool children through a mindfulness-based kindness curriculum. *Developmental Psychology, 51*(1), 44.

Good, C., Aronson, J., & Inzlicht, M. (2003). Improving adolescents' standardized test performance: An intervention to reduce the effects of stereotype threat. *Journal of Applied Developmental Psychology, 24*(6), 645–662.

Graziano, P. A., Reavis, R. D., Keane, S. P., & Calkins, S. D. (2007). The role of emotion regulation in children's early academic success. *Journal of school psychology, 45*(1), 3–19.

Haydicky, J., Wiener, J., Badali, P., Milligan, K., & Ducharme, J. M. (2012). Evaluation of a mindfulness-based intervention for adolescents with learning disabilities and co-occurring ADHD and anxiety. *Mindfulness, 3*(2), 151–164.

Hofmann, S. G., Sawyer, A. T., Witt, A. A., & Oh, D. (2010). The effect of mindfulness-based therapy on anxiety and depression: A meta-analytic review. *Journal of Consulting and Clinical Psychology, 78*(2), 169.

Hong, Y., Chiu, C., & Dweck, C. S. (1995). Implicit theories of intelligence. In *Efficacy, agency, and self-esteem* (pp. 197–216). Springer. Retrieved from http://link.springer.com/chapter/10.1007/978-1-4899-1280-0_10

Jensen, E. (1998). *Teaching with the brain in mind.* Association for Supervision & Curriculum Development. Retrieved from http://eric.ed.gov/?id=ed434950

Jha, A. P., Stanley, E. A., Kiyonaga, A., Wong, L., & Gelfand, L. (2010). Examining the protective effects of mindfulness training on working memory capacity and affective experience. *Emotion, 10*(1), 54–64. http://doi.org/10.1037/a0018438

Kabat-Zinn, J. (1990). *Full catastrophy living.* New York: Delta.

Kane, M. J., Brown, L. H., McVay, J. C., Silvia, P. J., Myin-Germeys, I., & Kwapil, T. R. (2007). For whom the mind wanders, and when: An experience-sampling study of working memory and executive control in daily life. *Psychological Science, 18*(7), 614–621. http://doi.org/10.1111/j.1467–9280.2007.01948.x

Killingsworth, M. A., & Gilbert, D. T. (2010). A wandering mind is an unhappy mind. *Science, 330*(6006), 932–932.

Kuyken, W., Weare, K., Ukoumunne, O. C., Vicary, R., Motton, N., Burnett, R., . . . Huppert, F. (2013). Effectiveness of the mindfulness in schools programme: Non-randomised controlled feasibility study. *The British Journal of Psychiatry, 203*(2), 126–131.

Leonard, N. R., Jha, A. P., Casarjian, B., Goolsarran, M., Garcia, C., Cleland, C. M., . . . Massey, Z. (2013). Mindfulness training improves attentional task performance in incarcerated youth: A group randomized controlled intervention trial. *Consciousness Research, 4*, 792. http://doi.org/10.3389/fpsyg.2013.00792

Levinson, D. B., Stoll, E. L., Kindy, S. D., Merry, H. L., & Davidson, R. J. (2014). A mind you can count on: Validating breath counting as a behavioral measure of mindfulness. *Frontiers in Psychology, 5*, 1201–1202. http://doi.org/10.3389/fpsyg.2014.01202

Lindquist, S. I., & McLean, J. P. (2011). Daydreaming and its correlates in an educational environment. *Learning and Individual Differences, 21*(2), 158–167.

MacLean, K. A., Ferrer, E., Aichele, S. R., Bridwell, D. A., Zanesco, A. P., Jacobs, T. L., . . . Saron, C. D. (2010). Intensive meditation training improves perceptual discrimination and sustained attention. *Psychological Science, 21*(6), 829–839.

Maynard, B. R., Solis, M., & Miller, V. (2015). *Mindfulness-based interventions for improving academic achievement, behavior and socio-emotional functioning of primary and secondary students: A systematic review.* Retrieved from http://campbellcollaboration.org/lib/download/3829/Maynard_Mindfulness_Protocol.pdf

Molden, D. C., & Dweck, C. S. (2006). Finding meaning in psychology: A lay theories approach to self-regulation, social perception, and social development. *American Psychologist, 61*(3), 192.

Mrazek, M. D., Franklin, M. S., Phillips, D. T., Baird, B., & Schooler, J. W. (2013). Mindfulness training improves working memory capacity and GRE performance while reducing mind wandering. *Psychological Science*, *24*(5), 776–781.

Mrazek, M. D., Mooneyham, B. W., Mrazek, K. L., & Schooler, J. W. (2016). Pushing the limits: Cognitive, affective, & neural plasticity revealed by an intensive multifaceted intervention. *Frontiers in Human Neuroscience*, *10*, 117.

Mrazek, M. D., Phillips, D. T., Franklin, M. S., Broadway, J. M., & Schooler, J. W. (2013). Young and restless: Validation of the Mind-Wandering Questionnaire (MWQ) reveals disruptive impact of mind-wandering for youth. *Frontiers in Psychology*, *4*. Retrieved from http://www.ncbi.nlm.nih.gov/pmc/articles/PMC3753539/

Mrazek, M. D., Phillips, D. T., & Schooler, J. W. (2015). *Mindfulness and theories of mind-wandering in high school freshman.* Preliminary Data, University of California, Santa Barbara.

Mrazek, M. D., Smallwood, J., Franklin, M. S., Chin, J. M., Baird, B., & Schooler, J. W. (2012). The role of mind-wandering in measurements of general aptitude. *Journal of Experimental Psychology: General*, *141*(4), 788–798. http://doi.org/10.1037/a0027968

Mrazek, M. D., Smallwood, J., & Schooler, J. W. (2012). Mindfulness and mind-wandering: Finding convergence through opposing constructs. *Emotion*, *12*(3), 442–450.

Nidich, S., Mjasiri, S., Nidich, R., Rainforth, M., Grant, J., Valosek, L., . . . Zigler, R. L. (2011). Academic achievement and transcendental meditation: A study with at-risk urban middle school students. *Education*, *131*(3), 556.

Risko, E. F., Anderson, N., Sarwal, A., Engelhardt, M., & Kingstone, A. (2012). Everyday attention: Variation in mind wandering and memory in a lecture. *Applied: Cognitive Psychology*, *26*(2), 234–242. doi:10.1002/acp.1814

Robins, R. W., & Pals, J. L. (2002). Implicit self-theories in the academic domain: Implications for goal orientation, attributions, affect, and self-esteem change. *Self and Identity*, *1*(4), 313–336.

Roeser, R. W., Schonert-Reichl, K. A., Jha, A., Cullen, M., Wallace, L., Wilensky, R., . . . Harrison, J. (2013). Mindfulness training and reductions in teacher stress and burnout: Results from two randomized, waitlist-control field trials. *Journal of Educational Psychology*, *105*(3), 787–804. http://doi.org/10.1037/a0032093

Rosengrant, D. (2011). Impulse-momentum diagrams. *The Physics Teacher*, *49*(1), 36–39.

Ross, M. (1989). Relation of implicit theories to the construction of personal histories. *Psychological Review*, *96*(2), 341–357. http://doi.org/10.1037/0033-295X.96.2.341

Sammons, P. (1995). *Key characteristics of effective schools: A review of school effectiveness research.* ERIC. Retrieved from http://eric.ed.gov/?id=ED389826

Schacter, D. L., & Szpunar, K. K. (2015). Enhancing attention and memory during video-recorded lectures. *Scholarship of Teaching and Learning in Psychology*, *1*(1), 60.

Schooler, J. W., Reichle, E. D., & Halpern, D. V. (2004). Zoning out while reading: Evidence for dissociations between experience and metaconsciousness. In D. T. Levin (Ed.), *Thinking and seeing: Visual metacognition in adults and children* (pp. 204–226). Cambridge, MA: MIT Press.

Semple, R. J., Lee, J., Rosa, D., & Miller, L. F. (2010). A randomized trial of mindfulness-based cognitive therapy for children: Promoting mindful attention to enhance social-emotional resiliency in children. *Journal of Child and Family Studies*, *19*(2), 218–229.

Shapiro, S. L., Brown, K. W., Thoresen, C., & Plante, T. G. (2011). The moderation of mindfulness-based stress reduction effects by trait mindfulness: Results from a randomized controlled trial. *Journal of Clinical Psychology*, *67*(3), 267–277.

Short, M. M., & Mazmanian, D. (2013). Perfectionism and negative repetitive thoughts: Examining a multiple mediator model in relation to mindfulness. *Personality and Individual Differences*, *55*(6), 716–721.

Smallwood, J., Fishman, D. J., & Schooler, J. W. (2007). Counting the cost of an absent mind: mind wandering as an underrecognized influence on educational performance. *Psychonomic Bulletin & Review*, *14*(2), 230–236.

Smallwood, J., Fitzgerald, A., Miles, L. K., & Phillips, L. H. (2009). Shifting moods, wandering minds: Negative moods lead the mind to wander. *Emotion (Washington, D.C.)*, *9*(2), 271–276. http://doi.org/10.1037/a0014855

Smallwood, J., McSpadden, M., & Schooler, J. W. (2008). When attention matters: The curious incident of the wandering mind. *Memory & Cognition*, *36*(6), 1144–1150. http://doi.org/10.3758/MC.36.6.1144

Smallwood, J., & Schooler, J. W. (2006). The restless mind. *Psychological Bulletin*, *132*(6), 946–958. http://doi.org/10.1037/0033–2909.132.6.946

Sylwester, R., & Cho, J.-Y. (1993). What brain research says about paying attention. *Educational Leadership*, *50*(4), 71–75.

Tang, Y. Y., Ma, Y., Wang, J., Fan, Y., Feng, S., Lu, Q., . . . Posner, M. (2007). Short-term meditation training improves attention and self-regulation. *Proceedings of the National Academy of Sciences*, *104*(43), 17152.

van de Weijer-Bergsma, E., Formsma, A. R., de Bruin, E. I., & Bögels, S. M. (2011). The effectiveness of mindfulness training on behavioral problems and attentional functioning in adolescents with ADHD. *Journal of Child and Family Studies*, *21*(5), 775–787. http://doi.org/10.1007/s10826-011-9531-7

Walburg, V. (2014). Burnout among high school students: A literature review. *Children and Youth Services Review*, *42*, 28–33.

Wammes, J. D., Seli, P., Allan, J., Boucher, P. O., & Smilek, D. (2016). Mind wandering during lectures II: Relation to academic performance. *Scholarship of Teaching and Learning in Psychology*, *2*(1), 33–48. http://doi.org/10.1037/stl0000055

Weare, K. (2013). Developing mindfulness with children and young people: A review of the evidence and policy context. *Journal of Children's Services*, *8*(2), 141–153.

Wine, J. (1971). Test anxiety and direction of attention. *Psychological Bulletin*, *76*(2), 92.

Yeager, D. S., & Dweck, C. S. (2012). Mindsets that promote resilience: When students believe that personal characteristics can be developed. *Educational Psychologist*, *47*(4), 302–314.

Yeager, D. S., & Walton, G. M. (2011). Social-psychological interventions in education: They're not magic. *Review of Educational Research*, *81*(2), 267–301.

Zanesco, A. P., King, B. G., MacLean, K. A., Jacobs, T. L., Aichele, S. R., Wallace, B. A., . . . Saron, C. D. (2016). Meditation training influences mind wandering and mindless reading. *Psychology of Consciousness: Theory, Research, and Practice*, *3*(1), 12.

Zedelius, C., Protzko, J., & Schooler, J. W. (2016). *Lay theories of mind wandering affect the rate of mind wandering in everyday life and in the lab*. Preliminary Data, University of California, Santa Barbara.

11

REDUCING SEPARATENESS WITH PRESENCE

How mindfulness catalyzes intergroup prosociality

Daniel R. Berry and Kirk Warren Brown

> Ultimately, peace is . . . about attitudes, about a sense of empathy, about breaking down the divisions that we create for ourselves in our own minds and our hearts that don't exist in any objective reality, but that we carry with us generation after generation.
>
> – President Barack Obama (2013)

Throughout history, intergroup conflict has had a devastating impact on societies and cultures, contributing to more than 200 million deaths in the 20th century alone (Cohen & Insko, 2008). At the heart of this issue, perceiving psychological separateness between "us" and "them" is psychological kindling for intergroup neglect, prejudice, discrimination, and full-blown aggressive conflict (Cikara, 2015; Zaki & Cikara, 2016). Social and political movements have inspired popular, scholarly, and scientific interest in ameliorating intergroup tension, and as a means to this end, social psychological approaches converge on identifying and cultivating psychological factors that bolster prosocial attitudes across social and cultural lines (see Batson & Ahmad, 2009 for review). Implicit to the promotion of prosocial attitudes and actions is the quality of attention paid to the person with whom one is interacting. Barrett-Lennard (1981) pointed out that an "empathic attentional set" is necessary for successful intergroup interactions, in which one "opens him- or herself in a deeply responsive way to another person's feelings" (p. 92).

How does one attend deeply to the other? Despite theoretical perspectives asserting the importance of attention in prosocial attitudes and action (e.g. Darley & Latané, 1970), little social psychological research has examined the role of attentional *quality* in these domains. *Mindfulness* offers particular promise in the study of intergroup prosociality, for several reasons. First, mindfulness entails a heightened capacity for careful – one could even say, *unconditional* – attention to internal and external stimuli from moment to moment. A growing body of research from the cognitive sciences indicates that gains in sustained attention, executive attention, and other indicators of well-functioning attention capacities accrue with mindfulness training (MT; Jha, Krompinger, & Baime, 2007; Slagter et al., 2007; Tang et al., 2007; van den Hurk, Giommi, Gielen, Speckens, & Barendregt, 2010). Second, there is initial indication that such training has positive social, including prosocial consequences (Condon, Desbordes, Miller, & DeSteno, 2013). Finally, training in mindful attention may be more transferable to social contexts than other attention training methods (Tang & Posner, 2009). Therefore, mindfulness provides a fitting lens through which to examine the role of attentional variation in intergroup prosociality.

The interpersonal benefits of mindfulness have been highlighted by the religious and philosophical traditions from which the concept and experience is derived, which emphasize the importance of disengaging from the often automatic, self-centred concerns that help to preserve the perceived psychological distance that separates "us" from "them" and thereby inhibit interpersonal sensitivity and meaningful connection with others (e.g. Brown, Berry, & Quaglia, 2016; Leary & Terry, 2012; Trautwein, Naranjo, & Schmidt, 2014). Consistent with this, a recent meta-analysis found a moderate effect size of MT on salutary interpersonal outcomes ($r = 0.44$; Sedlmeier et al., 2012). Drawing upon the centuries-old practice and more recent science of mindfulness, we propose in this chapter that the inherent receptivity of mindful attention helps to set the stage for prosociality across social and cultural lines.

In this chapter we focus on two consequences of group membership, namely defensive attitudes and reduced prosocial emotion and action toward out-group members. We discuss ways in which our and others' research indicates that mindfulness can attenuate these psychological states and behaviours. We will close by offering two potential mechanisms by which mindfulness may catalyze intergroup prosociality, namely de-automatization and dis-identification.

Mindfulness and defensive intergroup attitudes

Belonging to a cohesive social group has its benefits, not the least of which is that group membership is necessary to one's survival (Brewer & Caporael, 2006). Membership in cooperative groups allows for reciprocal exchange of food and other tangible resources, provides potential mates and protection from threat, and promotes the dissemination of cultural values and knowledge (De Dreu, Balliet, & Halevy, 2014). Furthermore, group membership fosters psychological and social well-being (e.g. Baumeister & Leary, 1995). Although the benefits of group membership are legion, feeling that one belongs to a group is typically accompanied by less willingness to cooperate with and help those who do not belong (Cikara, Bruneau, &

Saxe, 2011) and can even foster neglect of, and/or aggression toward social out-group members (Tooby & Cosmides, 2010).

As social beings, individuals are embedded within the broader worldviews of their social and cultural groups, these worldviews reflecting values, ideals, and beliefs about the world and the role of the individual and social groups within it. Common group identity valorizes in-group members, encourages reciprocal exchange and trust, and provides a source of shared meaning among members of the in-group (Pyszczynski, Greenberg, Solomon, Arndt, & Schimel, 2004) – but conflict and tension arise when this shared meaning is threatened or attacked. Contemporary and historical examples abound of individuals and groups aggressing against, neglecting, or derogating rival groups when they threaten in-group worldviews and social identity.

Contemplative theorists have long emphasized the potential for mindfulness and other meditation practices to bridge perceived gaps between self and other, us and them (e.g. Leary & Terry, 2012; Trautwein, Naranjo, & Schmidt, 2014). In this section we present nascent evidence that mindfulness fosters non-defensive attitudes toward social out-group members in three domains: worldview threat, linguistic intergroup bias, and automatic implicit bias.

Worldview threat

According to Terror Management Theory (TMT; Pyszczynski et al., 2004), annihilation of the self in death represents both a physical threat and symbolic threat to personal and social identity. Reflecting on one's death typically provokes anxiety, leading to efforts to manage this anxiety by defending social and cultural worldviews – both being symbolic representations of the self. Most commonly, worldviews are defended by favouring in-group and derogating out-group members to maintain a sense of permanence of one's self after certain death. Neimeic et al. (2010) asked whether mindful individuals, who are theorized to be less invested in identity, would show lower worldview defence in response to contemplating death. In a series of studies, those researchers created worldview threats after priming participants with an exercise making their own mortality salient. For example, in one study American citizens wrote either about their death or about watching TV (a control condition), and after a brief delay read scenarios that commonly evoke worldview defence (reading an essay by an anti- or pro-American peer). Compared to those lower in basic dispositional mindfulness, more mindful individuals evidenced less (in fact, almost no) derogation of the anti-American author and little favouritism toward the pro-American author. Similar results were found when considering a racial out-group member and a moral transgressor. Additional studies in the series showed that more mindful individuals did not simply distract from thoughts about death, but were more open to processing the threat, spending more time writing about their death and using more death-related words. This greater openness to processing mortality mediated the inverse relation between mindfulness and lower worldview defence. Consistent with the hypothesis that mindfulness reduces defensiveness toward out-group members, these studies showed that the tendency to bolster symbolic representations of the self under conditions of mortality salience was dampened.

Linguistic intergroup bias

The language that we use to describe others reveals our privately held beliefs and attitudes about them, implicitly transmitting stereotypic and prejudicial attitudes (Maass, 1999). Such beliefs are conveyed through linguistic abstraction that varies from concrete descriptions of others' behaviours ("person A struck person B") to abstract character judgements ("person A is violent"; Semin & Fiedler, 1992). When out-group members engage in positive actions that violate our stereotypic beliefs about them, people commonly make concrete verbal descriptions of those behaviours; in contrast, abstract character inferences based on group stereotypes are made when explaining negative actions of out-group members (Maass, 1999).

Tincher, Lebois, and Barsalou (2015) asked whether brief MT would dampen stereotypic and prejudicial attitudes, as reflected in attenuated linguistic intergroup bias. Participants were randomized to either brief MT or a control condition that involved absorption in vivid details of personal thoughts. After these exercises, participants were shown hand-drawn pictures depicting an individual engaged in a negative or positive behaviour (e.g. hitting or helping another person). Participants then chose one of four linguistic descriptions of the behaviour, ranging in degree of abstraction. For example, if shown a picture of an individual helping another person from the ground, choices ranged from (a) "Person A is picking up the other person" (concrete), (b) "Person A is helping the other person," (c) "Person A is concerned about the other person," and (d) "Person A is considerate" (abstract). Group status was manipulated by asking participants to imagine either their best friend (in-group) or worst enemy (out-group) engaging in these actions while making these judgements. Consistent with prior studies of linguistic intergroup bias (Maass, 1999), it could be expected that an in-group member (best friend) would be more frequently rated abstractly (e.g. "considerate") in positive contexts, whereas an out-group member (worst enemy) would be more frequently rated concretely (e.g. "picking up the other person") in positive contexts. The opposite pattern of results could be expected to occur for negative behaviours. The study showed, however, that MT participants evidenced less linguistic intergroup bias, as they chose fewer concrete linguistic descriptions of pictures depicting out-group members engaged in positive behaviours and fewer abstract linguistic descriptions of pictures depicting out-group members engaged in negative behaviours. Thus, brief MT prior to intergroup judgement reduced the tendency to choose language perpetuating stereotypic and prejudiced thinking.

Automatic implicit bias

Implicit attitudes are based on automatic associations between two or more constructs in memory (Greenwald & Banaji, 1995). Coming into contact with a representative of a social group for which a stereotype schema is present automatically activates attitudes about them (e.g. Devine, 1989), and these attitudes have a number of often-unintended consequences detrimental to intergroup interactions, ranging from discriminatory hiring decisions (Rudman & Glick, 2001), to more frequent shooting of ambiguously threatening out-group members (Correll, Park, Judd, & Wittenbrink, 2002). Growing research interest in the contemplative science community on attenuating implicit bias has sparked systematic study of the effects of mindfulness and other meditation practices on implicit attitudes. Kang, Gray, and Dovidio (2014) demonstrated that non-Black adults receiving 6-week loving-kindness meditation (LKM) training, relative to those in a loving-kindness discussion group, showed reduced implicit bias against Blacks and the homeless, as measured by the Implicit Association Test (IAT; Greenwald, McGhee, & Schwartz, 1998). Stell and Farsides (2015) found that among White participants even brief (10-min) LKM afforded lower automatic activation of, and greater conscious control over implicit racial biases against Black individuals on the IAT. The researchers found that positive emotions toward the out-group mediated the effect of LKM on implicit racial bias reduction.

The meditation training in these studies was multimodal in form, including directing participants in how to be more sensitive toward others, but there is evidence that a mindful state itself reduces implicit bias. Lueke and Gibson (2014) asked whether deploying mindful attention could reduce implicit race and age biases. Participants were randomized to receive a brief (10-minute) mindfulness induction or a matched control induction prior to completing the race and age IAT. Results showed that MT decreased implicit race and age bias, presumably because mindfulness weakened automatically activated associations on the IAT.

Together, these studies of worldview defence, explicit linguistic bias, and implicit bias show a consistent pattern of non-defensiveness toward out-group members, and a profile of intergroup interaction that begins with open or receptive presence toward the other. In the next section we turn to evidence showing that mindfulness can also foster kindness toward social out-group members.

Mindfulness and intergroup prosociality

When predicaments befall others, humans express an innate and learned capacity to empathize with them and to show them kindness and care (de Waal, 2008). Perhaps in part because seeking and maintaining long-lasting social relationships is a basic psychological need (Deci & Ryan, 1985), empathy is often expressed unintentionally, and even toward strangers (Preston & de Waal, 2002). Contemporary examples abound, however, of people failing to help others in need. Decety and Chaminade

(2003) suggest that before empathic responses can be made, a person in need must first be perceived to be like or similar to a prospective helper. Although most people condemn discrimination and endorse egalitarian attitudes, intergroup contexts are frequently marked by an "empathy gap" in which prosociality is often lacking (e.g. Cikara et al., 2011).

As stated earlier, mindfulness has been theorized to help close the psychological distance between self and others (e.g. Condon, Chapter 9 in this volume; Trautwein et al., 2014). If mindfulness fosters disengagement from self-centred concerns (Feldman, Greeson, & Senville, 2010), then it may also enhance the perceived similarity between self and others more readily than as compared to states of self-absorption or inattentiveness to automatic attitudes that arise in intergroup interactions. Thus, if prosocial emotion and action are promoted by perceived similarity, mindfulness could be expected to foster prosociality in intergroup contexts.

Mindfulness in intergroup prosocial emotion and action

Prosocial emotions and actions crucially begin with careful attention to the person in need (Darley & Latané, 1970). Although implicit to theories of prosociality, quality of attention is a largely overlooked determinant of prosocial emotion and action. But in interpersonal contexts attention is a nuanced phenomenon, requiring attention to the present situation so as to notice the person's predicament and also "tuning in" to one's own internal somatic and affective responses to that situation (Singer, Critchley, & Preuschoff, 2009). This interoceptive awareness is particularly important in the generation of empathy, as individuals rely on such awareness to simulate the affected person's mental and emotional state, drawing upon their own prior mental and emotional experiences of similar circumstances (Gallese & Goldman, 1998). MT has been shown to enhance interoceptive awareness (Bornemann, Herbert, Mehling, & Singer, 2014), and consequently, empathy and helping behaviour toward strangers (Berry et al., 2016b; Condon et al., 2013; Lim, Condon, & DeSteno, 2015), who are often shown fewer kindnesses than shown toward "known" others. If, as Desbordes et al. (2015) theorize, mindfulness is characterized by unconditional, equanimous attention, its prosocial benefits should extend to intergroup interactions. In this section we present nascent research from our lab showing that mindfulness fosters prosocial emotion and action to strangers and other out-group members.

In three experiments by Berry, Brown, and Cairo (2016a) participants were randomized to listen to either a brief (10-minute) audio-recorded MT, a structurally equivalent attention training, or to receive no instruction, and then witnessed a person with a dissimilar personality (Study 1) or race (Studies 2–3) being ostracized or excluded in an online ball-tossing game (Cyberball; Williams, Yeager, Cheung, & Choi, 2012). Relative to those in the control conditions, MT participants reported higher empathic concern for the victim (and lower empathic anger toward the perpetrators). MT participants also wrote more comforting emails to the victim and included them more often during a later "all play" Cyberball game. Empathic concern mediated the effect of MT on helping behaviour outcomes, suggesting that a state of mindful attention fostered more empathy and subsequently, more helping behaviour.

Berry et al. (2016a) extended these findings to *in vivo* social interactions by implementing scenario-based indicators of helping behaviour. Self-identifying Caucasian White participants were randomized to receive one of the two following scenarios: (1) the experimenter ostensibly accidentally dropped a large stack of informed consent documents on the floor, or (2) another ostensible participant walked into the waiting room on crutches and leaned uncomfortably against the wall (cf., Condon et al., 2013). The race of the confederate needing help (White or Black) was also randomized. Thereafter participants completed a series of self-report measures including a commonly used measure of basic dispositional mindfulness (Brown & Ryan, 2003) and a measure of racial prejudice toward African Americans (Henry & Sears, 2002). Although there were no differences in the frequency of helping toward same-race versus other-race confederates in need, more mindful individuals helped more often in both scenarios. Further, while self-reported racial prejudice predicted less helping in the interracial conditions, dispositional mindfulness qualified this relation, such that more-mindful individuals helped more frequently regardless of their racial attitudes toward African Americans. Together, these studies provide initial support for the positive role of mindful attention in intergroup prosociality.

Kind presence: how mindfulness may reduce separateness

As these incipient lines of research develop, the question arises as to why mindfulness conduces to less defensiveness and greater prosociality toward out-group members. In this section we suggest that mindful attention can help to override automatic mental processes that foster separateness, and can encourage social responses absent a strong overlay of self-identification, offering greater potential for choiceful action. Through these mechanisms, we suggest, mindfulness is thought to foster kind action toward others, including out-group members, without presupposition as to their traits, intentions, goals, or worldviews.

De-automatizing separateness

The capacity to be mindful stands in stark contrast to much of our daily experience, in which we operate on automatic pilot without much awareness of what we are doing (Bargh & Chartrand, 1999). We easily drift off into mind-wandering (Killingsworth & Gilbert, 2010), and when provoked or stressed, we often act and react automatically (e.g. Kang, Gruber, & Gray, 2013). In states of automaticity, awareness operates in service to automatic thoughts, feelings, desires, and behaviours.

Mindfulness is thought to allow a clear, moment-to-moment glimpse into what one is thinking, feeling, or doing, in which events are "seen" without dominance by conceptual thought (Olendzki, 2005). This mindful stance allows one to notice mental processes as they arise, or to notice the psychological effects of those processes on one's experience and behaviour, and then slow, interrupt, change, or override these automatic cognitions, emotions, and behaviours. Levesque and Brown (2007) demonstrated that for those lower in basic dispositional mindfulness, implicit autonomy orientation was significantly positively associated with day-to-day autonomous motivation; more mindful individuals, however, showed higher day-to-day autonomous motivation regardless of implicit autonomy orientation. These results indicate that among those lower in implicit autonomous orientation, mindfulness tempered the unconscious tendency to associate the self with low volition. These findings are consistent with mindfulness theory in showing that a predisposition toward this state of mind was associated with less automatized, more choiceful behaviour on a day-to-day basis.

More germane to the present exposition, perceiving separateness between "me" and "them" or "us" and "them" can occur automatically. As previously stated, mere exposure to a member of a social category (based on race, sex, political orientation, etc.) activates schemas based on the stereotypic traits, intentions, and behaviours of that out-group (e.g. Devine, 1989), and this categorization process innervates downstream intergroup prejudice, neglect, and conflict (Billig, 1985). These processes, however, can be controlled and/or overridden (Devine & Sharp, 2009). For example, increasing awareness of one's prejudiced attitudes and behaviours can attenuate their expression (Banaji, Bazerman, & Chugh, 2003). Thus, heightening awareness to intergroup cognitions, emotions, and interactions via mindful awareness may afford more choiceful responses that are less constrained by automatic intergroup biases.

Further, mindfulness may promote a lessening of stereotypic and prejudicial attitudes, particularly as a consequence of long-term MT. Devine, Forscher, Austin, and Cox (2012) suggest that interventions that aim to reduce intergroup biases typically cultivate awareness of those biases as a first step toward reducing them. In this way, MT could create a disposition in which frequent awareness of one's own stereotypic and prejudiced responses in intergroup interactions serves to reduce them altogether.

Dis-identification: breaching interpersonal separateness

Self-identification with a social category or group is a necessary first step toward in-group favouritism and intergroup conflict. Tajfel (1981) defines such identification as "the part of an individual's self-concept which derives from his knowledge of his membership of a social group together with the value and emotional significance attached to that membership" (p. 255). Brewer (2001) states: "social identification involves affective and evaluative processes that are above and beyond cognitive classification. The affective significance arises from the felt attachment between the self and the in-group" (p. 21). Only when one incorporates the group into one's personal and social identity do intergroup tensions arise. Social Identity Theory posits that individuals are motivated to enhance and maintain self-esteem by achieving positive in-group distinctiveness: the tendency to perceive one's social in-group as *distinct* from and *better* than other out-groups (Tajfel, 1982). Even among individuals assigned to "minimal groups" that are created on an arbitrary basis (in the lab, for example), distinctions are made between "us" and "them" and are especially exaggerated when they favour the in-group (Tajfel, 1978). Favouring one's in-group(s) promotes positive interactions among in-group members, but can also have downstream consequences that are detrimental to the harmony of intergroup relations: "Privileging members of our group, by correlation, de-privileges those who do not belong to it" (Ricard, 2015, p. 277). Out-group members are perceived as homogenous, and we often neglect their psychological complexity, relying on cognitive shortcuts about their traits, goals, intentions, and behaviours to inform the social interaction (Park & Judd, 1990).

Personal and social identities are dynamic constructs that involve identification with particular attributes, roles, group memberships, and worldviews that are consistent with appraisals that one has made over time (Gilbert, 2005). The lay view of identity entails that one maintains a coherent and consistent view of the self that is separate from others (Metzinger, 2003). Interpersonal and intergroup interactions can be viewed as interactions between self-representations of those individuals that are mediated by and filtered through each person's internalized views of self and other (Leary, 2002). When mindful attention is brought to self-representations and other thoughts as they arise, change, and fade away, the ephemeral nature of such processes can be "seen," affording a dis-identification with them (Brown et al., 2016; Brown et al., 2008).

Through both mechanisms briefly discussed here – namely reduced automaticity and relative self dis-identification – we suggest that mindfulness may lead to less emotional reactivity to identity threats, greater understanding and acceptance of social group differences, and ultimately more harmonious intergroup interactions. In so doing, mindfulness may promote the kinds of altered cognitive, emotional, and overt behavioural responses discussed in this chapter, including lessened stereotyping, prejudice, and discrimination, lower identification-driven conflict and neglect of out-group members, and higher levels of prosocial action.

Conclusions and further considerations

This chapter highlighted findings supporting the theory that mindfulness facilitates adaptive intergroup interactions, which are particularly expressed in lower defensive behaviour and increased prosociality across social and cultural lines. The research presented herein is promising, but more well-controlled experimental research that pits MT against active control conditions is required to better understand whether and why mindfulness fosters positive intergroup interactions. Addressing these questions necessitates an examination of the various forms that MT can take. At present it is unclear which forms of training – for example, in open monitoring, focused attention, or loving kindness (compassion) – are most valuable for cultivating intergroup harmony.

What psychological mechanisms drive the positive intergroup consequences of mindfulness? In this chapter we proposed two potential reasons why mindfulness has such effects, namely that this state of mind is comparatively less subject to automatic intergroup biases, and promotes psychological states and behaviour marked by less self-identification (i.e. is "hypo-egoic"; Brown & Leary, 2016; see also Leary & Diebels, Chapter 4 in this volume). Other mechanisms are plausible as well; for example, intergroup prosociality could also be supported by the purported emotion regulatory advantage of mindfulness (Arch & Landy, 2015). Social psychological and social neuroscience approaches to empathy suggest that one must regulate one's own negative affect to an affected person's predicament prior to helping them (Decety & Jackson, 2004), and mindfulness may offer emotion regulatory benefits in such circumstances.

All of the research presented here focused on individual-level psychological and behavioural outcomes in intergroup contexts. Researchers ought to be cognizant of the group and societal level antecedents and consequences of mindfulness as well. Interest in the positive consequences of mindfulness practice for national well-being has reached the political realm (Ryan, 2012).

What are the adaptive implications for mindfulness in intergroup prosociality? We have emphasized the adaptive nature of mindfulness, but might it have adaptive costs to the individual and/or group? For instance, intergroup conflict is often rife with unfair and unjust treatment of individuals for which empathic anger might energize confrontation to cease injustices (Vitaglione & Barnett, 2003). We found that brief MT conduced to lower empathic anger toward perpetrators after witnessing social exclusion and did not predict punishment of perpetrators (Berry et al., 2016b). Another study found that those higher in dispositional mindfulness were significantly less likely to intervene in an intergroup bullying scenario (Berry et al., 2016c). Righteous anger and punishment are only one way to confront injustice, and historical examples abound of individuals using compassionate, non-violent means to halt social injustices. Mindful attention appears to catalyze similar responsiveness that is focused on ameliorating victim suffering, rather than correcting or punishing perpetrators of unfair and unjust acts.

We hope this chapter invites further research to better comprehend the role of mindful attention in intergroup contexts. As this line of inquiry develops it will also be important to understand how to best apply the basic research findings to promote *in vivo* positive intergroup and cross-cultural interactions. While many agree that people should be sensitive to others regardless of their racial, national, and other social group memberships, the real challenge is to know it "in one's bones." Perhaps, as has been suggested for millennia, we will discover that by looking inside ourselves to investigate our own human proclivities, we become kinder and more compassionate – because underneath the surface differences, we recognize the commonality of experience that all people share.

References

Arch, J. J., & Landy, L. N. (2015). Mindfulness and emotional benefits. In K. W. Brown, J. D. Creswell, & R. M. Ryan (Eds.), *Handbook of mindfulness: Theory and research* (pp. 208–224). New York: Guilford Press.

Banaji, M. R., Bazerman, M. H., & Chugh, D. (2003). How (un)ethical are you? *Harvard Business Review, 81*(12), 56–64.

Bargh, J. A., & Chartrand, T. L. (1999). The unbearable automaticity of being. *American Psychologist, 54*(7), 462. doi:10.1037/0003-066X.54.7.462

Barrett-Lennard, G. T. (1981). The empathy cycle: Refinement of a nuclear concept. *Journal of Counseling Psychology, 28*, 91–100. doi:10.1037/0022-0167.28.2.91

Batson, C. D. & Ahmad, N. Y. (2009). Using empathy to improve intergroup attitudes and relations. *Social Issues and Policy Review, 3*, 141–177. doi:10.1111/j.1751-2409.2009.01013.x

Baumeister, R. F., & Leary, M. R. (1995). The need to belong: Desire for interpersonal attachments as a fundamental human motivation. *Psychological Bulletin, 117*(3), 497–529. doi:10.1037/0033-2909.117.3.497

Berry, D. R., Brown, K. W., & Cairo, A. H. (2016a). The inherent kindness of presence: Brief mindfulness training catalyzes prosocial responses across social lines. Unpublished manuscript, Virginia Commonwealth University, Richmond, VA.

Berry, D. R., Brown, K. W., Cairo, A. H., Goodman, R. J., Quaglia, J. T., & Green, J. D. (2016b). Mindfulness increases empathic and prosocial responses toward ostracized stranger. *Journal of Experimental Psychology: General.*

Berry, D. R., Griffin, B. G., Garthe, R., Davis, D. E., & Worthington, E. (2016c). Dispositional mindfulness is associated with reduced bully intervention. Unpublished manuscript, Virginia Commonwealth University, Richmond, VA.

Billig, M. (1985). Prejudice, categorization and particularization: From a perceptual to a rhetorical approach. *European Journal of Social Psychology, 15*(1), 79–103. doi:10.1002/ejsp.2420150107

Bornemann, B., Herbert, B. M., Mehling, W. E., & Singer, T. (2014). Differential changes in self-reported aspects of interoceptive awareness through 3 months of contemplative training. *Frontiers in Psychology, 5*, 1504. doi:10.3389/fpsyg.2014.01504

Brewer, M. B. (2001). Ingroup identification and intergroup conflict. In R. D. Ashmore, L. Jussim, & D. Wilder (Eds.), *Social identity, intergroup conflict, and conflict reduction* (pp. 17–41). New York: Oxford University Press.

Brewer, M. B., & Caporael, L. R. (2006). An evolutionary perspective on social identity: Revisiting groups. In M. Schaller, J. A. Simpson, & D. T. Kenrick (Eds.), *Evolution and social psychology* (pp. 143–161). New York: Psychology Press.

Brown, K. W., Berry, D. R., & Quaglia, J. T. (2016). The hypo-egoic expression of mindfulness in social life. In M. L. Leary & K. W. Brown (Eds.), *The Oxford handbook of hypo-egoic processes.* New York: Oxford University Press.

Brown, K. W., & Leary, M. R. (2016). The emergence of scholarship and science on hypo-egoic phenomena. In K. W. Brown & M. R. Leary (Eds.), *The Oxford handbook of hypo-egoic phenomena* (pp. 3–16). New York: Oxford University Press.

Brown, K. W., & Ryan, R. M. (2003). The benefits of being present: Mindfulness and its role in psychological well-being. *Journal of Personality and Social Psychology, 84*(4), 822–848. doi:10.1037/0022-3514.84.4.822

Brown, K. W., Ryan, R. M., Creswell, J. D., & Niemiec, C. P. (2008). Beyond me: Mindful responses to social threat. In H. A. Wayment & J. J. Bauer (Eds.), *Transcending self-interest: Psychological explorations of the quiet ego* (pp. 75–84). Washington, DC: American Psychological Association.

Cikara, M. (2015). Intergroup schadenfreude: Motivating participation in collective violence. *Current Opinion in Behavioral Sciences, 3*, 12–17. doi:10.1016/j.cobeha.2014.12.007

Cikara, M., Bruneau, E. G., & Saxe, R. R. (2011). Us and them: intergroup failures of empathy. *Current Directions in Psychological Science, 20*(3), 149–153. doi:10.1177/0963721411408713

Cohen, T. R., & Insko, C. A. (2008). War and peace: Possible approaches to reducing intergroup conflict. *Perspectives on Psychological Science, 3*(2), 87–93. doi:10.1111/j.1745-6916.2008.00066.x

Condon, P., Desbordes, G., Miller, W., & DeSteno, D. (2013). Meditation increases compassionate responses to suffering. *Psychological Science, 24*(10), 2125–2127. doi:10.1177/0956797613485603

Correll, J., Park, B., Judd, C. M., & Wittenbrink, B. (2002). The police officer's dilemma: Using ethnicity to disambiguate potentially threatening individuals. *Journal of Personality and Social Psychology, 83*(6), 1314. doi:10.1037/0022-3514.83.6.1314

Darley, J. M., & Latané, B. (1970). *The unresponsive bystander: Why doesn't he help?* New York: Appleton Century Crofts.

Decety, J., & Chaminade, T. (2003). When the self represents the other: A new cognitive neuroscience view on psychological identification. *Consciousness and Cognition, 12*(4), 577–596. doi:10.1016/S1053-8100(03)00076-X

Decety, J., & Jackson, P. L. (2004). The functional architecture of human empathy. *Behavioral and Cognitive Neuroscience Reviews, 3*(2), 71–100.

Deci, E. L., & Ryan, R. M. (1985). *Intrinsic motivation and self-determination in human behavior.* New York: Plenum.

De Dreu, C. K., Balliet, D., & Halevy, N. (2014). Parochial cooperation in humans: Forms and functions of self-sacrifice in intergroup conflict. *Advances in Motivation Science, 1*, 1–47. doi:10.1016/bs.adms.2014.08.001

Desbordes, G., Gard, T., Hoge, E. A., Hölzel, B. K., Kerr, C., Lazar, S. W., . . . Vago, D. R. (2015). Moving beyond mindfulness: Defining equanimity as an outcome measure in meditation and contemplative research. *Mindfulness, 6*(2), 356–372.

Devine, P. G. (1989). Stereotypes and prejudice: Their automatic and controlled components. *Journal of Personality and Social Psychology, 56*(1), 5–18. doi:10.1037/0022-3514.56.1.5

Devine, P. G., Forscher, P. S., Austin, A. J., & Cox, W. T. (2012). Long term reduction in implicit race bias: A prejudice habit-breaking intervention. *Journal of Experimental Social Psychology, 48*(6), 1267–1278. doi:10.1016/j.jesp.2012.06.003

Devine, P. G., & Sharp, L. B. (2009). Automaticity and control in stereotyping and prejudice. In T. D. Nelson (Ed.), *Handbook of prejudice, stereotyping, and discrimination* (pp. 61–87). New York: Psychology Press.

de Waal, F. B. (2008). Putting the altruism back into altruism: The evolution of empathy. *Annual Review of Psychology, 59*, 279–300. doi:10.1146/annurev.psych.59.103006.093625

Feldman, G., Greeson, J., & Senville, J. (2010). Differential effects of mindful breathing, progressive muscle relaxation, and loving-kindness meditation on decentering and negative reactions to repetitive thoughts. *Behaviour Research and Therapy, 48*(10), 1002–1011. doi:10.1016/j.brat.2010.06.006

Gallese, V., & Goldman, A. (1998). Mirror neurons and the simulation theory of mind-reading. *Trends in Cognitive Sciences, 2*(12), 493–501. doi:10.1016/S1364-6613(98)01262-5

Gilbert, P. (2005). *Compassion: Conceptualisations, research and use in psychotherapy.* New York: Routledge.

Greenwald, A. G., & Banaji, M. R. (1995). Implicit social cognition: Attitudes, self-esteem, and stereotypes. *Psychological Review, 102*(1), 4–27. doi:10.2307/1129610

Greenwald, A. G., McGhee, D. E., & Schwartz, J. L. (1998). Measuring individual differences in implicit cognition: The implicit association test. *Journal of Personality and Social Psychology, 74*(6), 1464–1480. doi:10.1037/0022-3514.74.6.1464

Henry, P. J., & Sears, D. O. (2002). The symbolic racism 2000 scale. *Political Psychology, 23*(2), 253–283.

Jha, A. P., Krompinger, J., & Baime, M. J. (2007). Mindfulness training modifies subsystems of attention. *Cognitive, Affective, & Behavioral Neuroscience, 7*(2), 109–119. doi:10.3758/cabn.7.2.109

Kang, Y., Gray, J. R., & Dovidio, J. F. (2014). The nondiscriminating heart: Lovingkindness meditation training decreases implicit intergroup bias. *Journal of Experimental Psychology: General, 143*(3), 1306–1313. doi:10.1037/a0034150

Kang, Y., Gruber, J., & Gray, J. R. (2013). Mindfulness and de-automatization. *Emotion Review, 5*(2), 192–201. doi:10.1177/1754073912451629

Killingsworth, M. A., & Gilbert, D. T. (2010). A wandering mind is an unhappy mind. *Science, 330*(6006), 932–932. doi:10.1126/science.1192439

Leary, M. R. (2002). The interpersonal basis of self-esteem: Death, devaluation, or deference? In J. P. Forgas & K. D. Williams (Eds.), *The social self: Cognitive, interpersonal, and intergroup perspectives* (pp. 143–159). New York: Psychology Press.

Leary, M. R., & Terry, M. L. (2012). Hypo-egoic mindsets: Antecedents and implications of quieting the self. In M. R. Leary & J. P. Tangney (Eds.), *Handbook of self and identity* (pp. 268–288). New York: Guilford Press.

Levesque, C., & Brown, K. W. (2007). Mindfulness as a moderator of the effect of implicit motivational self-concept on day-to-day behavioral motivation. *Motivation and Emotion, 31*(4), 284–299.

Lim, D., Condon, P., & DeSteno, D. (2015). Mindfulness and compassion: An examination of mechanism and scalability. *PLoS ONE, 10*(2), e0118221.

Lueke, A., & Gibson, B. (2014). Mindfulness meditation reduces implicit age and race bias: The role of reduced automaticity of responding. *Social Psychological and Personality Science, 6*(3), 284–291. doi:10.1177/1948550614559651

Maass, A. (1999). Linguistic intergroup bias: Stereotype perpetuation through language. *Advances in Experimental Social Psychology, 31*, 79–122. doi:10.1016/S0065-2601(08)60272-5

Metzinger, T. (2003). Phenomenal transparency and cognitive self-reference. *Phenomenology and the Cognitive Sciences, 2*(4), 353–393. doi:10.1023/B:PHEN.0000007366.42918.eb

Niemiec, C. P., Brown, K. W., Kashdan, T. B., Cozzolino, P. J., Breen, W. E., Levesque-Bristol, C., & Ryan, R. M. (2010). Being present in the face of existential threat: The role of trait mindfulness in reducing defensive responses to mortality salience. *Journal of Personality and Social Psychology, 99*(2), 344.

Obama, B. H. (2013, June 17). Remarks by President Obama and Mrs. Obama in town hall with youth of Northern Ireland. Retrieved from https://www.whitehouse.gov/the-press-office/2013/06/17/remarks-president-obama-and-mrs-obama-town-hall-youth-northern-ireland

Olendzki, A. (2005). The roots of mindfulness. In C. K. Germer, R. D. Siegel, & P. R. Fulton (Eds.), *Mindfulness and psychotherapy* (pp. 241–261). New York: Guilford Press.

Park, B., & Judd, C. M. (1990). Measures and models of perceived group variability. *Journal of Personality and Social Psychology, 59*(2), 173–191. doi:10.1037/0022-3514.59.2.173

Preston, S. D., & De Waal, F. B. (2002). Empathy: Its ultimate and proximate bases. *Behavioral and Brain Sciences, 25*(1), 1–20. doi:10.1017/S0140525X02000018

Pyszczynski, T., Greenberg, J., Solomon, S., Arndt, J., & Schimel, J. (2004). Why do people need self-esteem? A theoretical and empirical review. *Psychological Bulletin, 130*(3), 435–468. doi: 10.1037/0033-2909.130.3.435

Ricard, M. (2015). *Altruism: The power of compassion to change yourself and the world.* New York: Atlantic Books.

Rudman, L. A., & Glick, P. (2001). Prescriptive gender stereotypes and backlash toward agentic women. *Journal of Social Issues, 57*(4), 743–762. doi:10.1111/0022-4537.00239

Ryan, T. (2012). *A mindful nation: How a simple practice can help us reduce stress, improve performance, and recapture the American spirit*. New York: Hay House.

Sedlmeier, P., Eberth, J., Schwarz, M., Zimmermann, D., Haarig, F., Jaeger, S., & Kunze, S. (2012). The psychological effects of meditation: A meta-analysis. *Psychological Bulletin, 138*(6), 1139–1171. doi:10.1037/a0028168

Semin, G. R., & Fiedler, K. E. (1992). *Language, interaction and social cognition*. Thousand Oaks, CA: Sage.

Singer, T., Critchley, H. D., & Preuschoff, K. (2009). A common role of insula in feelings, empathy and uncertainty. *Trends in Cognitive Sciences, 13*(8), 334–340. doi:10.1016/j.tics.2009.05.001

Stell, A. J., & Farsides, T. (2015). Brief loving-kindness meditation reduces racial bias, mediated by positive other-regarding emotions. *Motivation and Emotion, 40,* 140–147.

Tajfel, H. E. (1978). *Differentiation between social groups: Studies in the social psychology of intergroup relations*. Oxford: Academic Press.

Tajfel, H. E. (1981). *Human groups and social categories: Studies in social psychology*. New York: Cambridge University Press.

Tajfel, H. E. (1982). Social psychology of intergroup relations. *Annual Review of Psychology, 33*(1), 1–39.

Tang, Y. Y., Ma, Y., Wang, J., Fan, Y., Feng, S., Lu, Q., ... Posner, M. I. (2007). Short-term meditation training improves attention and self-regulation. *Proceedings of the National Academy of Sciences, 104*(43), 17152–17156. doi:10.1073/pnas.0707678104

Tang, Y. Y., & Posner, M. I. (2009). Attention training and attention state training. *Trends in Cognitive Sciences, 13*(5), 222–227. doi:10.1016/j.tics.2009.01.009

Tincher, M. M., Lebois, L. A., & Barsalou, L. W. (2015). Mindful attention reduces linguistic intergroup bias. *Mindfulness, 7,* 349–360.

Tooby, J. & Cosmides, L. (2010). Groups in mind: The coalitional roots of war and morality. In H. Høgh-Olesen (Ed.), *Human morality and sociality: Evolutionary and comparative perspective* (pp. 191–234). London: Palgrave Macmillan.

Trautwein, F. M., Naranjo, J. R., & Schmidt, S. (2014). Meditation effects in the social domain: Self-other connectedness as a general mechanism? In S. Schmidt, & H. Walach (Eds.) *Meditation–neuroscientific approaches and philosophical implications* (pp. 175–198). Heidelberg: Springer International.

van den Hurk, P. A., Giommi, F., Gielen, S. C., Speckens, A. E., & Barendregt, H. P. (2010). Greater efficiency in attentional processing related to mindfulness meditation. *The Quarterly Journal of Experimental Psychology, 63*(6), 1168–1180. doi:10.1080/17470210903249365

Vitaglione, G. D., & Barnett, M. A. (2003). Assessing a new dimension of empathy: Empathic anger as a predictor of helping and punishing desires. *Motivation and Emotion, 27*(4), 301–325. doi:10.1023/A:1026231622102

Williams, K. S., Yeager, D. S., Cheung, C. K. T., & Choi, W. (2012). *Cyberball (version 4.0)* [Software]. Retrieved from https://cyberball.wikispaces.com

Zaki, J., & Cikara, M. (2016). Addressing empathic failures. *Psychological Science, 24*(6), 471–476. doi:10.1177/0963721415599978

INDEX